Life in the Fast Lane

Stephany Alleyroux

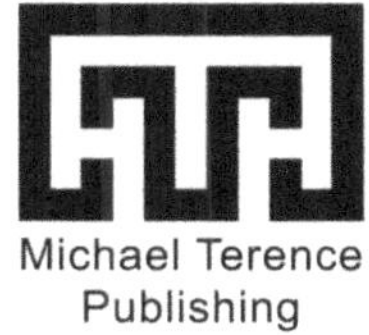

Michael Terence
Publishing

First published in paperback by
Michael Terence Publishing in 2019
www.mtp.agency

ISBN 9781912639601

Life in the Fast Lane

Stephany Alleyroux

Contents

Foreword

I have been hopeful about one-day offering advice on something I am familiar with, as well as about sharing my success story. A small introduction won't hurt, right?

My name is Stephany Alleyroux. I am 21 years of age, a personal assistant, student and I also help run my mother's business 'Glitzy Candles & Accessories', and now I am also a published author.

I became open about my sugar dating experience in 2018 and how well it had worked out for me, resulting in a wonderful long-term relationship. I count myself as blessed and fortunate to have met a man as amazing as he is, and we both look forward to seeing what the future holds for us. I know our future will be great. I'd love to be able to help someone find a man or woman suited to them as well.

I've experienced so many wonderful times during my time sugar dating, such as going on extravagant holidays and short trips, receiving designer gifts and luxury items, being financially supported and being mentored when necessary.

Our whirlwind romance started the minute we met, and that can happen to you too! Love doesn't see how long it has been, how you met or anything for that matter, it just happens. As unbelievable as it may sound to you, sugar dating can lead to that love.

No matter what it is that you're looking for, be it a strict sugar daddy/mummy-sugar baby fling, a serious relationship with sugar benefits or just a more conventional relationship, there will be something in this book for you! I'll be shedding some light as to how both men and women can find exactly what they're looking for. I'm here to guide both sugar babies as well as sugar daddies or sugar mommies to get what they want; so, I hope you're sitting comfortably because you're in for a ride!

1: Who Are You? What to Expect

First thing's first, you should know that this is not a formal book. Think of it as more like a conversation with a friend, confidante or mentor. However, the only difference will be that we won't be directly communicating, in fact, you'll be soaking in information directly from the pages and asking yourself the questions I will put forward for you to mull over.

I am a firm believer in 'no money, no happy relationship or marriage'. I do not believe that one can be happily married to someone and be poor. Sorry, but I'm not sorry. It might sound superficial but hear me out for a second to understand my perspective. As soon as there is no money or less money coming in, notice that it is when problems come in, and the bickering starts.

To put it simply, if you have no money, do not get into a serious relationship or get married. This might not sit well with some people, but the reality isn't always pretty. If the breadwinner in a household suddenly stops bringing in bread, problems are bound to occur. The same goes for the homemaker; if a homemaker doesn't look after the home and family, then problems and arguments will arise. Each person plays a certain role in their relationship and there is nothing wrong with that.

I'm <u>NOT</u> saying break up with someone if they stop

making money or they stop doing their relationship 'requirements' because if you truly love someone, you will work it out with them <u>BUT</u> it certainly will put a strain on the relationship whether you stick together or not. This strain will give rise to bitterness, regardless of how many times you try to cover it up or lie to yourself. Money matters lead to bitterness and bitterness is unhealthy for a relationship, which is my point.

Sugar dating simply makes it easier to establish who will be playing what role and how can both parties please each other without any extra headaches. Also, sugar dating allows more clarity as both partners know where they stand and what they need to do to keep the other person happy. There are no confusions; there is just transparency.

There seems a stigma attached to sugar dating, which is that such a relationship is between a beautiful young lady and a rich older man. That can certainly be the case, and it is the most common type of sugar couple. However, there are more people now who sugar date, despite not fitting into this stereotype. Different kinds of people are searching for different things which bring us down to the most popular misconception attached to this – sugar dating is not just about money or sex. Sugar dating is not a selfish arrangement where one or both partners take advantage of each other. In fact, sugar dating is free of exploitation, and false hopes and promises.

The reality is that there are young men dating elder

women. There are single mums looking for some support. There are middle-aged women looking for someone around their own age that they can just settle down with. There are young women like myself who have met an established man, have a bright future with him, have formed a solid relationship and are in it for the long run. There are people looking for less conventional relationships, short term, long distance, online arrangements, and the possibilities go on!

Sugar dating is fun, it's easy and everyone is looking for something so it is mostly a judgement free zone. Everyone is able to lay their cards on the table without holding back or receiving any backlash for what they want.

Do not ever be ashamed of using sugar daddy websites as the means of finding somebody. If it works for you, then that is all that matters and nobody else should have a say. So, let's move onto how to get started in the sugar dating world.

Let's start with sugar babies. You must ask yourself, "who am I?", "what are my goals?" and "what have I experienced in life so far?". Yes, I'm very serious. The most important thing to remember is that nobody is going to help you if you don't help yourself. That includes a sugar daddy/mummy or boyfriend/girlfriend. Ideally, you'll be a student, have a job or be active in pursuing your career. You'll need to be passionate about something and have goals! Your sugar daddy/mummy or boyfriend/girlfriend will find that very attractive as you won't just be a pretty face.

spoiler alert Rich men/women can find beautiful women/men ANYWHERE so make sure that you stand out!

Your other half may be so invested in you that they might help you reach your goals or to advance in whatever field you're passionate about.

Next step is fashion sense and looks. I know this and so do you that looks matter a lot. Shallow and predictable much? However, it is the key factor that initially attracts potential partners. This step comes before getting to know someone so both ladies and gentlemen need to bring in their A-game. You need to invest in yourself. Do not neglect the hair, skin and nails ladies! Get those open toe shoes you were looking at and wear them with pride because your pedicure is done!

As for men, wear a nice crisp white shirt on your date with some good aftershave will do the trick also keeping that trim fresh (unless you're bald then you have no cause for concern) because as women, we like our men to look presentable.

Now this part applies to both parties, but mainly to sugar daddies and sugar mummies. STANDARDS. Everyone always thinks about their standards are and rightly so. Settling for less than your worth is never an option but keep it realistic. Your blessings may lie with someone that isn't your usual type. We are part of the social networking generation, which includes online dating! Remember to be open minded. The fundamental factors that are not up for negotiation are:

- Good hygiene – If the person generates a foul odour. LEAVE and never look back. They're too grown up for someone to have to tell them to wash.
- Good manners and respect – The sugar dad or sugar mummy is not an ATM. The sugar baby is not a piece of meat. Keep that in mind.

With all good things comes changes. Whether you make the most of it or not, is up to you. The best place to meet is usually Central London. There is a vast amount to do there. You could go to restaurants, wine or cocktail bars, even sight-seeing or shopping. A great playfield also for those who tend not to date online. Many people from all different and interesting backgrounds visit Central London; so ladies get your group together and go out for a few drinks, you may meet some lovely gentlemen. Go out and explore what the beautiful city has to offer! You'd be surprised.

Your lifestyle and habits will change once you begin to sugar date. Especially when you find someone you plan to be with. Be prepared for that change. You may need to become more flexible with time or even with where you are based.

2: Introduction to Websites

Where it all started for me was on a sugar daddy website, RichMeetBeautiful® to be precise. Now, it's important to realise that not all websites cater to the same audience.

When joining a website, you must ask yourself what it is that you are looking for. Some sites will have more people looking for things like pay per meets or hook-ups. Some will have the majority looking for a no strings attached sugar daddy (SD)/sugar mummy (SM) – sugar baby (SB) situation. Others will provide people genuinely looking for a relationship with sugaring benefits or just your typical conventional relationship.

I found my relationship with sugaring benefits on RichMeetBeautiful®, which worked out great for me. There is a good ratio of men and women out there from all over the world. I'd recommend this site to anyone who is considering sugar dating. It is straightforward, hassle-free and great filtering options.

Once you find the website you'd like to join, it'll be time to create a profile. Keep in mind that you do not have to join a sugar daddy site to sugar date. You also do not have to join a mainstream dating website to date 'normally'. It is entirely up to you as long as you make your intentions clear. However, it is much easier to date on a website that is accommodating to what you are looking for. You can, for example, change your preferred age range and tweak your bio.

Now, I've been asked countless of times what a person should put in a profile so pay attention. Firstly, don't post any pictures with Snapchat filters. Show your face. Show a nice full-length body picture, maybe even one of you on holiday would be nice. Blur out anyone else who is in the picture with you as they're entitled to their privacy. You should talk about what your profession and hobbies are. Maybe even character traits, but try not to sound too self-involved. Ladies, avoid using words like 'spoiled', 'princess', and any cheesy one-liners. Gentlemen, try not to sound too formal or forcibly funny in your bio. Arrogance shines brightly through bios too so sounding cocky or too big for your own boots won't work in your favour. Try to include anything exciting you've done or countries you have recently visited. Next, you should put what you would like to find in a person and on the site. Keep it short and sweet as you'll have time to further discuss options in your chats.

I understand that finding your match can be challenging, as there are millions of profiles. It is a bit like trying to find gold when there are many gold-plated items around. However, I kid you not, it is possible! You will talk to many men or women before finding someone who is suitable. Do not get discouraged. It is all part of the process after all. You may go through a few trial and errors before finding 'the one'. You also have to distinguish someone who is being genuine with you or someone who is simply feeding you a load of crap. This is one of the reasons why it is so important to stay grounded and not setting your expectations too high. He or she will take care of you and trust them on that.

You've got to ask yourself what it is that you are seeking from the site? There are many different types of relationships you can gain from sugaring. For example, pay per meets (PPM), no strings attached (NSA), strictly sugar daddy/mummy and sugar baby, a relationship with the sugaring benefits, a conventional relationship, just to name a few.

I'll elaborate...

Pay per meets (PPM) –the sugar daddy or sugar mummy will give you money (usually in cash) every time the two of you decide to meet. What you do during this time is at your discretion. This type of arrangement usually is non-monogamous.

No strings attached (NSA) – similar to pay per meets, but the cash may not be exchanging hands every time you meet. This means while it may have relationship benefits, there will be no official label or commitment. Both parties are free outside of this arrangement to do whatever they choose to do. It usually is non-monogamous and there is no string attached.

Strictly sugar daddy/mummy and sugar baby – this is more exclusive than the NSA arrangement though still without an official title. It may mean only seeing each other once or twice in a month. The SD/SM may have done this before and if so, it may run more smoothly because they know what they are doing and what will be in the SB's best interest. Having a previous SB prior to the arrangement will allow the potential slow start to speed up. This arrangement is usually monogamous though some do prefer to have more than one sugar baby. Some sugar babies prefer to have two or more sugar daddy/mummies at one time. With this can come money, gifts, holidays, among other luxuries.

Relationship with sugaring benefits – this will be completely exclusive. The pair will be in a conventional relationship with added benefits. This may include, but not limited to, gifts, money, holidays, and more. It can even develop into such as marriage if the love develops between them. Everything feels genuine. (This best describes my relationship).

Conventional relationship – it is quite common to see people looking for a conventional relationship on a sugaring website. This will have no specific additional bonuses but will also be completely exclusive. May include a few trips away like couples usually do.

Be prepared to have offers such as cuckolding and being the third addition to a relationship. It often happens but if it's not for you, then politely decline. There may even be men who offer money in exchange for domination. There are many things that you can explore.

On the site you choose, you'll be presented with a few options such as liking a profile, sending them some kind of wink or even being able to initiate a conversation. These are the initial ways to filter as you get to decide whom you'd like to be better acquainted with. You must make sure to READ THE PROFILE. I can't stress that enough. The profile allow you to learn more about the person you're interested in. It's no use judging a person solely on the basis of their looks because the two of you may be on different wavelengths. Save yourself days of wasted time by just reading a profile. Looking at pictures is great but reading the profile gives you some valuable insights, which will help you enormously when starting up a conversation.

There will be a filtering process no matter what outcome you're looking for.

The filtering process is to eliminate anyone who doesn't want the same things as you, isn't someone you can see yourself with whether it's because of their looks, the way they've expressed what they want or simply that the two of you have different ideas about what they want to find in a person or a relationship. You'll have the option to narrow down your search. Some sugar dating websites give more options than others do, but in general, they help to keep your focus on what you'd like.

Keep an eye out for people who have been on the website for a long time. What is their reason? Have they deactivated their account and only recently re-joined? Are they a serial dater? Potential time waster? Or just picky? It is important to know before initiating contact.

If you are thinking, 'what should I look out for in a SD/SM?' then look no further!

I've made a little **should have/do and shouldn't have/do's** list for you.

Your SD/SM **should have/do's**;

A profession – a good one at that. Find out more about it. You may find someone who can introduce you to some great opportunities.

Good heart/understanding/compassionate – having a SD/SM that isn't kind hearted, will just not work.

A clear understanding of what you would like in your arrangement/relationship – this one is actually the most important one. Before getting involved with each other, your SD/SM should know everything you'd expect so there are no surprises down the line. If they are happy with it and you are happy with theirs, the two of you will be able to move forward.

Time – your SD/SM should make time for you at the very least twice a month if your arrangement/relationship is an offline one.

A sense of humour/something in common with you; it just makes life easier.

Your SD/SM **should** form an amazing bond with you. Maybe even love if it's something more serious.

Be a joy to be around – some SD/SM's may be quite reserved but does not mean they aren't fun to be around. Will be even better if they're not so bad on the eyes too. Being happy to be seen around with them is quite necessary if that's what it will involve. In my case, I love to be out with my man.

Your SD/SM **shouldn't have/do's**;

Multiple SBs – nobody wants to share the person they're with unless it is agreed upon. Your SD/SM should let you know if you are not the only SB they have or if they're involved with someone else as well (married or otherwise).

Active profiles – once the two of you are officially involved, ALL PROFILES MUST BE DELETED. That includes yours.

Bad hygiene – because nobody should smell bad.

Your SD/SM **should not** waste your time.

Try to stay realistic in terms of what you are looking for. As much as a £5,000 a month allowance with no strings attached sounds very appealing, it is highly unlikely to happen. Sorry about that.

Try to keep it simple. To tell you the truth, I had no 'arrangement' with my boyfriend. It has always been spur of the moment, spoiling, and care. It feels more natural that way; it is how a relationship should feel. However, if a relationship is not what you are looking for then discussing a realistic arrangement is essential so that the two of you know exactly what you are setting yourselves up to, though not before starting up that conversation.

Ladies, do NOT be scared of starting the conversation, whether you're a sugar mummy or sugar baby. It's always sexy to go after what you want, or in this case, who you want. Just keep your options open. Do not risk everything on one endeavour before finding whom you have been searching for. Once you know, make sure to be invested and making that work.

3: How to Approach

What should you say when you start up a conversation?

NO TEXT TALK! Type correctly, it won't go unnoticed. Abbreviations for things such as 'laugh out loud (LOL) are okay, but we are grown adults. Introduction is everything. Saying "hi" or "how are you?" is too common and quite frankly very boring. This isn't a friend that you're catching up with. Beware of copied and pasted messages too. All messages sent and received should be personalised to fit the person you are talking to. This is someone you are trying to impress. Make yourself sound interesting and if anything in the persons profile peaks an interest, use it after you introduce yourself. Use it to your advantage, as it's something the two of you have in common. It also allows the other person to know that you've taken your time and carefully read through their profile. It will set you apart from those who don't care enough to read. I'm telling you, it goes a long way.

Reminder: some people will click 'favourite' on your profile and not talk. I personally would not indulge in their game of kiss chase. In saying that, if you like how they look or even their profile then humour them. Often what happens is they have gone on a 'liking' spree and will pick the best out of the bunch so make sure to stand out when sending them a message. This applies to everyone.

I would also like to be realistic, not everyone that you are attracted to will be attracted to you. You may be

ignored, blocked, speak to someone and they'll disappear. Do not allow it to affect you! Not everybody is like that. Also, some members haven't paid their membership so can't actually respond. Membership fees usually apply to the SD/SM. It applies to the SB on very few websites.

The following is relevant to sugar babies but concerns all.

Now that you have made contact, the conversation will gradually (sometimes immediately) turn to what you are looking for. Here, you'll need to explain what you'd like from them or what you'd like to experience with them. I will give you certain dating examples.

For PPM: here you may explain that you'd like to meet several times a month, maybe for lunch and you may take it further after. The sugar daddy/mummy will ask how much you'll be expecting. Here you'll need to give a price for each time you meet. A set amount of money. Remember that PPM won't involve gifts so think carefully. Analyse your situation carefully and see if the amount you request or are offered is suitable for you.

For NSA: you may see your sugar daddy/mummy more often than those in a PPM. This will have a more casual feel to it. You'll need to discuss what kind of NSA it will be. Will it feel like a relationship or not? Will money be a factor? Is it company you'd like? Trips away? Dinner dates? You can have many options here but remember not to do anything that'll allow you to develop deep emotions for the person.

For strictly SD-SM/SB: for this arrangement, an allowance is the most popular option. It can be monthly (most common choice) or weekly. The amount may vary depending on what else the SD/SM is offering. If travelling, gifts, and other luxuries are a part of the arrangement, there may be a lower allowance offered or none at all. It is up to the both of you to decide what works best for you. Do not be disheartened if the amount offered is not high, as it could increase over time or you'll be happy with the 'package deal'. It is important not to be greedy. A SD/SM is there to enhance your lifestyle and not to fund all of your activities. 'The best is yet to come' as they say.

Relationship with benefits -- as it's a relationship and speaking from personal experience, I would not start with talking about money at all. You can however, let him or her know that you'd like a relationship that will involve living your best life and experiencing new things and new places. That you'd also like to be spoiled from time to time. The level of 'spoiling' will differ in people so find someone who is on the same page as you. Your other half will know what that means and you can now focus on building a rock-solid relationship and spoil each other at the same time! It'll feel so natural that you'll both want to do more effort for the other person in any way possible. It's important to establish the trust and bond. Once that has been set in stone, you may let each other know what more you'd like aside from what you've already established.

I often am asked: "How do I get what you have?" and all I can say is that no two relationships are the same because everyone is different so you won't have the exact relationship that I have. I have found someone that would give me the world in an instant and I would do the same but that is because of how we complement each other.

What you can have is your own fulfilling relationship in its own way with someone that makes you happy and complements you. That is exactly what you will find!

This section is relevant for everyone!

This part of sugar dating catches many out as many people waste their time or don't find the right match. So... How do you know whether the person you're talking to is genuine?

Well... there are a number of things that you can do to make sure that you find the person with the right intentions.

First, A blank profile is never good. So, avoid profiles which do not contain much information about the person.

Secondly, if there is no picture, it doesn't necessarily means that it's a fake profile, but if they're not willing to send any pictures or share their private pictures with you, something is definitely not right there hunty.

If you begin to exchange words and eventually exchange numbers, then make sure to at the very least have a phone call. Texting each other is not enough! If they keep putting off the phone call, cancel them!

Try to communicate via video call, it's always nice to interact with someone that you are about to meet. It is a much safer way to talk before meeting as you've seen them before.

Another tip: Set a date to meet and DO NOT DELAY. I wouldn't wait more than three weeks and that's only if there's a date set. Do not allow the person to prolong the initial meet. My boyfriend and I couldn't meet for a few weeks initially but we had a date set and we stuck to it.

If the man or woman you are meeting is abroad, make sure that your tickets are booked soon otherwise it'll be a waste of time. My boyfriend lives abroad and my tickets are always booked. Do not allow them to waste your time. That goes for both parties.

You'll need to talk about what you both expect from each other – if they dodge the conversation then ABORT MISSION.

If money or sex constitutes the most part of your conversations, then it's a RED FLAG – there should be more to it than that. Even for the PPM.

Ask many questions – bombard them. It is the best way to get to know someone.

To end this chapter with some clear-cut advice, ladies/gentlemen, make sure that you do not come across as money hungry. The man or woman knows why you've joined. No need to mention it in every sentence. When the time comes to talk about finances, do so and move on from it.

To the SD/SMs', do not falsify what you have to offer. You'll only be wasting your own time.

Tip: SD/SM/your boyfriend may give you money for different reasons. Whether it is to help with bills, car payments, or just to treat you. It is easy to misuse that money and you may be left with nothing, yet again needing more. So, here is what you need to do, when you receive money, invest it or save it. Truth be told, you should be paying your own bills before they come along but I understand that times can really be hard. Sometimes making ends meet is difficult. So, if money is involved in the equation, you can put the money that they give towards future bills so you can have a little left over for yourself and rest assured knowing you have taken care of your priorities. If you love to shop like I do then buy items that hold their value. There are smart ways to utilise what you are being given. Prioritise with what you have. Invest into the future. I'm not saying do not use the money for fun, by all means go right ahead but do so once you have sorted out your priorities. You do not want to rely on someone for life so be smart!

4: Meeting

Once you find the person you feel most connected to, there will come a time (hopefully soon after) that the two of you meet.

Planning to meet can be a nightmare sometimes. Certain factors can interfere and potentially create obstacle in something that could be great.

So, what to do when planning to meet someone?

It's essential to have two things to help with the process;

A passport to travel. Not having a passport can really affect what can happen between you and your other half if it's more than just PPM and if one person really loves to travel or does so for work.

Another thing is a full driver's licence. Though it may not be the most necessary thing, knowing how to drive even if you do not own a car can benefit you in many circumstances. If you go to visit your SD/SM/SB or boyfriend, and they are out for the day, the last thing you want is to be stuck indoors because you can't drive.

Despite the fact that most SD/SMs' financially support their SB when necessary, it is important to still be independent and not have to rely on them for everything. Having the two of these things sorted out will show that you still can stand on your own two feet. That's another attractive feature.

Reminder: your SD/SB/boyfriend is there to help and support you, love and nurture you as you do the same, yes. But you should help yourself as they are helping you. Don't just live your life based on what they give you.

Understanding that people can get busy is crucial when sugar dating. Your SD/SM will most likely be the busier one compared to you so learn to understand if the rendezvous cannot happen in the days or the week following. This will especially applicable to those who need to travel to a different country to see one another. These things may take some time, but not too much time. It is all about valuing the time of each other and not prolonging the date and time when you shall meet.

For the SD/SMs' out there, this means that you do not get a pass on wasting the SB's time. They also have a routine that they will take a break from to see you. SB's if your SD/SM is wasting your time, move on! Nobody has time for that.

The two of you will need to then establish what you'll be doing when you meet. If you are meeting up in London, I suggest going into central London. There is so much to do out there! 'if you're bored of London then you're bored of life' so get going! You can go to upmarket restaurants, posh bars, and different exciting places. During the winters, there's Winter Wonderland and much more to enjoy. You could go shopping; attend an event together or do anything else. You name it and London has it! It'll also be fun to explore together. As someone who resides in London, there are so many parts of it that I have yet to see so I'd strongly advise to be dolled up and go off on an adventure together.

If either of you is based abroad or even in a different city, one of you will need to commute (both of you if you are meeting somewhere in-between).

Living in a different city is cost effective and saves time. Find a place where you both will be comfortable. Try to avoid a noisy restaurant or a busy time of the day. There is nothing worse than shouting to get the other person to hear you or having too many distractions around. You're meant to be the centre of attention that day! That goes for both SD/SM and SBs'.

Going abroad is exciting, however! New country, new people and so many wonderful things to experience. Do the tourism tours! It'll be a fun bonding session. Incorporate some shopping for souvenirs to bring back with you. Whoever your host is (SD/SM/SB), make sure you feel at ease with them BEFORE booking any tickets. As for the host, ensure that you create a safe and enjoyable environment for whomever you're bringing with you. Should things not work out for the two of you, it is important to keep things amicable for the duration of their stay. Remain cordial. If things do work out, then great! Plan to meet up again!

Ladies; what to wear/pack?

For a weekend: Bring your essentials. Around two pairs of

heels. One of a nude tone and one black. I know it's tempting to bring your entire wardrobe, but you must resist the urge.

Bring your makeup kit but only the bare necessities. I say this because unless he is your boyfriend, sitting for two hours waiting on someone to do their makeup can be rather painful.

Clothes – make sure to bring a nice dress for an evening out, but keep the rest rather smart casual. To avoid packing too many clothes, bring the ones that mix and match.

Reminder: most European countries have loads of cobbles on their pavements and everything is usually in walking distance so flat shoes will be your best friend!

Five days or more: You may need a larger suitcase for this one, ladies! Still, keep it rather simple and do not over pack. Chances are you'll be doing some shopping wherever you are heading.

Bring your essentials, maybe your curling iron, a minimum of 7-outfits and make sure you can mix and match. About four pairs of shoes and some jewellery.

A bikini or swimsuit may be necessary and do not forget things such as adaptors and sun lotion.

I'm sure if you do forget anything, the person you are with will be rather accommodating. My boyfriend has been an absolute angel in that respect.

Having an itinerary can be helpful so you don't waste your days together doing the bare minimum. Do as much as you can in the days that you have together. There is only so much you'll have to say to each other just lazing around on the sofa all day long so keep things interesting! It also makes for good conversation when the two of you later reflect. You do not need to plan every second of everyday, but having an idea about what each day will involve will make life easier.

Meeting your potential or already established partner, (I'll use the word 'partner' because it can mean anything from somebody you are dating to someone that you are in a relationship with) can be such an exciting time. No matter if it's your first or 1000th time seeing them. The rush and the feelings remain the same (for me anyway). It is especially true when you do not get to see each other every day. It is like constantly going on a first date with the person you enjoy spending time with and/or love. You'll get to continuously do something exciting and even when you do have downtime together and do nothing, it'll still feel just as good just because you are together and enjoying each other's company.

I have had and am still having such wonderful experiences and have felt such adoration. It honestly is a true blessing to find someone with an amazing heart. Finding someone you'd do anything for was something I wasn't sure I'd find but I did and so did he. Okay, gushing is over and now coming back to the facts!

Your situation or arrangement will affect what happens when and where you meet. It'll especially impact how often you meet. The more serious or committed you are about each other, the more you'll be seeing each other. I suggest working out how your schedules fits together on a monthly basis and see where to go from there. You may find that you'll arrange to see each other last minute. Most of my trips abroad with my boyfriend were planned at the last minute. My trips to go over and see him are 97% of the time booked the day before. There are times when I cancelled my plans that I had lined up and sometimes call in sick for work. Oops! It is all about balancing and prioritising. My boyfriend will also move around business meetings to be able to see me or I'll travel with him even if he has to work on the trip. When you don't get to see them as much as you'd like to, make the most of the time that you do get with them. These are the moments you'll get to make a lasting impact on one another.

Something important to remember, especially for those dating someone much older than they are; your partner is most likely going to have children. You cannot be selfish with time and you have to be understanding when they may not be able to see you or are sometimes unable to communicate with you. You are free to express your take on the situation if you feel neglected, but be wary not to push your partner away. Kids may be their first priority.

If you are the one with children, make sure to split your time evenly or explain how often you'll be able to communicate with them and see them. Do not allow your partner to be in the dark. Should you slip up and keep your partner on the back burner or make them feel like they're not even on your list of priorities, it is your duty to reassure them that everything between the two of you is absolutely fine and throw in a few apologies for being absent or not paying as much attention. **This is especially applicable to those who are in a committed relationship.** It won't always be easy but if the person you are with is worth it, the two of you will work through anything.

Now, the taboo topic. **A married man or woman.** I am not one to judge and the simple fact is married people do join these sites mostly when they are lacking something in their marriage. Dealing with a married person will have its challenges. Some say it's wrong, some couldn't care less.

Be aware of what you are getting yourself into. Most married men and women that date will not be open to getting a divorce. Some married men/women have started their separation and divorce journey. If your partner is still very much involved with their family, make sure they let you know. In this case, I would not advise that it be anything more than PPM/NSA/strictly SD/SM/SB as developing feelings could result in something very messy.

If your partner is open to getting a divorce or is getting one, you could take it one step further and develop a relationship. I would advise to wait until he is a divorcee to avoid any complications.

For those that are married and are starting something serious, think about what you really want out of the relationship and communicate that with them. Do NOT mislead them and do NOT waste the other person's time.

Make sure to treat them well so they know that you do want to be with them. If you are only after a fling then make that clear too.

Reminder: this will be a delicate matter for everyone involved and while I wouldn't advise it, if you do find yourself in this situation, tread very carefully and take everyone's feelings into account. Some people genuinely fall in love with someone else when they are married or fall in love with someone who is married. How you decide to handle it can only be up to you. Just make sure that everyone involved is being treated as right and as fairly as can be.

To sum it up for you people, enjoy the company of the person you are with no matter where in the world it is in and no matter what you do!

5: Keeping Your Match Satisfied

Moving on to the more advanced stages now. This is really where the fun begins because at this stage, you'll be placing a lot of your time and energy into whoever you're with.

This chapter of my book will focus on how to keep your match interested and satisfied so that you can incorporate it in your own life. This applies to any form of relationship.

When you begin to speak to your partner, sometimes you give too much too quickly and they lose interest. It's important to sometimes hold back to stay mysterious and interested. If they know absolutely everything there is to know or you've given them everything they were interested in too fast, they may not stick around and that works both ways. Sometimes take a step back and see how the person reacts. Fight or flight. Will they stay or will they immediately say "screw this, I'm out"? Give a little out about yourself at a time. Remain interesting to the person. Do not become dull, a wet blanket or someone who spends their time complaining. Remember, this is meant to be a positive, potentially life changing experience. You will ruin it for yourself if you keep putting a damper on things.

After a while, the two of you will become more acquainted, you'll know more about each other, habits, likes, dislikes, etc. It may all become a little boring, so how do you keep one another interested? Get ready guys and girls! Here comes the fun part;

Stay sexy – works both ways. Keep yourself looking and smelling good each time you see your partner.

Get involved – join in on activities that you both enjoy or that the other person can teach you. Usually sporty activities with another person is a great bonding strategy. You can really become close and get to know each other on a deeper level. Maybe help with part of their business or help your partner get ready and organised for a certain project. Feeling artistic? Visit showrooms and museums together. The two of you will have so much to talk about and you'll both be in your element. Does one person love something in particular like dancing perhaps? Book a class! The person will appreciate it. Football? Get some tickets (to the right game people)! Shopping? Take her! It is also another bonding experience, believe it or not.

Tease – now, the more comfortable you get with each other, you will become more trusting of the other person. It's not to say that you must or should send any nude pictures of yourself. Everyone has a preference. Maybe involve some tempting words. Say something that will have the person wanting to drive or fly over to you that second!

Maybe a little teaser picture with no nudity necessary. Talk about something that has happened between the two of you before that had the sparks flying and passion building. The memories can be a big turn on for the both of you.

Allow the teasing to blend right into your quality time together. Wear something cute and sexy. Lingerie perhaps? Feed him/her fruit or use your hands and tongues on each other. Get sensual. Best of all? Smell good. Ladies, I recommend the Chanel Mademoiselle Intense or any of the Chanel perfume for that matter and for the men, I recommend Bleu de Chanel or Dior Sauvage.

Intellectual conversation – let the other person know how work is going. How your day has been, what has happened. If you need to vent a little then do so! The person will feel good knowing you trust them enough with this information (don't go on all day however, nobody wants to get their violins out). Take an interest also in their profession. Ask them various questions, how their day was, what they have coming up, work, and gossip even! Ask them whom they get along with at work. Do they have any big projects coming up? I'm sure you get the point. You can talk about business ideas that you have, a new business opportunity that you have. Your partner should be your biggest cheerleader and support system. They may even give you more ideas on how to improve your current plan or be able to put one in action for you.

Family – if the person has kids then take an interest. Ask them how their children are. It takes nothing to ask and it goes a long way. If anyone in their family is unwell or not in the right mind frame, make sure to check up on your partner and be there for them. Be that shoulder that they can cry on. When family celebrations are coming up, congratulate them! If you can't be a part of the day for whatever reason, be sure to still be supportive. Be the positive energy that they need.

General conversation – you don't need to talk all day, every day but checking up on someone can really brighten up their day so go ahead and do it. Make sure that the two of you bounce off each other and that there is good banter. Nothing is worse than being around someone and their energy is off or jokes aren't funny.

Honesty – please, PLEASE be transparent with each other when it comes to things you like or don't like. This includes but is not limited to:

Personality traits - are they kind? Short tempered? Bad with responses? Good with affection? Whatever the case may be, let your partner know. Praise them or say it's something you both need to work on.

Likes - is there anything in particular that they do that you enjoy? Is the sex good? What can be improved? Is there anything you'd both like to try out? BDSM? Involving someone else? Different locations? Fantasies. Do not be shy when it comes to talking about this. Are they kind? Their looks? Their scent? The way they hold you? LET THEM KNOW!

Dislikes - arrogance? Ignorance? Cocky? Is there something he or she does in the bedroom that need to stop? Hygiene? How do they treat others? Be honest with each other so you can decide if you make a good pair or not.

Be open to trying new things together to keep things interesting whether it's in or out of the bedroom. Be kind and know how to treat them.

Another factor that keeps it interesting (for me anyway) is not constantly seeing each other. Give each other some space, time to miss one another. When you see each other again, there will be so much raw emotion and it is awesome! Stay in touch over the phone by all means, but keep that spark between you. Keep the person excited to see you. You may buy yourself some kinky lingerie ladies or he may do it for you. Gentlemen, you may plan something really nice for the two of you. Do not be afraid to be romantic. Book that last-minute flight, the table reservation and a nice hotel with a view. You'll see how well that works out for you. Thank me later!

This will give the two of you something to look forward. A build-up of sexual frustration, lust, and love. You want to crave the affection and experience of being with the other person. That is when you know you are on a good path together.

The best thing to keep in mind is just to be more open to new ideas and try new things, explore different places with each other. No experience is the same.

This section is directed towards female readers and male SBs:

As women, sometimes we feel as though making the first move or being the one to make more of an effort is bad. I'm here to tell you that it's not a bad thing at all. With everything you wish to keep, you must take care of. Your partner is no different. Start the conversation every now and then; prove that you are interested. You'll gain nothing by acting too laid back or disinterested. If he feels as though you have no interest, he or she will move on right along to someone else who is prepared to constantly and consistently show their passion, appreciation, care and love. It should not always be the man making the first steps. Show interest, keep things spicy between the two of you and he will have eyes for no other. Total investment in you. For some of you your man or woman will be the 'provider' so to speak. This means you have to step your game up and bring something to the table. Making him or her feel amazing and appreciated is the least that you can do.

This section is directed towards male readers who are SDs:

Naturally, as a man who has joined as a SD, you will be making many kind gestures. You will be putting your gentleman's hat on and impressing your lady. I'm rather traditional. I believe that a man should look after the woman he is with, as should she, but in different ways. Gentlemen, keep your woman happy and she will be on her bended knee asking you to marry her (Kidding but you get the point). The effort works both ways. Just because you may be the provider does not mean you can purposely neglect other elements. We like to feel wanted, loved, cared for, and cherished. All of these things are important to women.

I'm going to include in this chapter also what tolerance level you should have. It goes hand in hand with how to keep someone interested and satisfied.

What should or shouldn't you tolerate from the man or woman that you are with?

I'll do this in two parts.

Starting with sugar babies – your SD/SM will have some requirements of their own. You'll need to be accepting of those or you need to find someone else.

Under no circumstances should you deal with someone who treats you like a sex object.

Do not allow anybody to speak to you as if you are beneath them; they joined the site looking for something too!

If you feel like he or is she playing you or being dishonest, then ask.

If your think that they are wasting your time e.g. no phone calls, date to meet or you are waiting a day or more for a response, block and delete that person.

If you'd prefer to be exclusive but they do not, then do not settle.

These are the basic and fundamental rules. However, you can set more for yourself or can even decide to tolerate a few of these.

As for the SD/SMs':

Do not allow the sugar baby to treat you like an ATM. You have agreed to help and spoil them, but to the limit that the two of you set together.

Do not allow the sugar baby to dictate how you should spend your finances. You stick to the agreement that was set and go the extra mile if that's what you feel is right.

You should set your boundaries i.e. discretion.

This is something for both the SD/SM and SB – DO NOT LET THEM PRESSURISE YOU. You are free to make any decision that you like.

6: For the Sugar Daddies

This chapter will focus on the sugar daddies and the sugar mummies out there! The majority of this book so far has been directed towards the sugar babies but I can't forget about you guys!

I'll be covering different questions or dilemmas that you may have.

The main objective of a SD/SM is to find someone to distract them from the 'real' world. To have some company without the stress of life and just to be able to enjoy some hassle-free time whilst bringing something to the table that they can benefit from. But, how do you know if he or she is the right SB for you?

You may all have different ideas about what you'd like your sugar baby to be like especially when it comes to appearance, so I will not cover that too much. What I will put out there is to stay realistic. The same way a SB shouldn't expect hundreds or thousands of pounds a month. A SD/SB should also be realistic in what they can attain. Believe it or not, a SB can be just as choosy as you decide to be, so do not be too picky. There are many balls in everybody's court. Nobody has the upper hand in the sugaring world unless you give it to them.

There are a few basic **should have/do's**;
Your SB **should** have a profession or should be a student.

Your SB **should** carry themselves well in public. After all, they'll be a representation of you.

Your SB **should** be on the same page as you. No use having a SB that has a completely different idea of how things are going to work and unfold.

Your SB **should** have things in common with you. What else will you talk about?

Your SB **should** be willing to learn from you, allow you to guide them and introduce them to new and exciting opportunities/people/places.

Your SB **should** be carefree – having someone who brings out the best in you is always a bonus in my book!

Your SB **should** make you feel comfortable doing things you never thought you would!

Your SB should benefit in all kinds of ways from being with you and having you around as you should with them.

Your SB should bring you out of your shell!!! This is such an important factor. The two of you should not be bored of each other. He or she should always be a joy to be around. Maybe even your arm candy – nothing wrong with that. I'm my boyfriend's arm candy and proud of it. He loves to flaunt me around and I never disappoint.

There are also a few basic should not/do's;

Your SB **should not** rely on you for every single expense. SORRY SB'S! But, it's true, use the money your SD/SB gives you wisely so you won't be broke!

Your SB **should not** be disruptive. Set the boundaries.

Everyone should know where they stand.

Your SB **should not** be a source of stress. They should be a positive person in your life.

Your SB **should not** go against your initial agreement unless the both of you have agreed upon a change.

Your SB **should not** be moody – we all have our bad days, which is acceptable, but bad days should not be every day nor should they affect your every day.

Your SB **should not** have multiple SD/SM's unless you have agreed on that he or she can.

If you have been unlucky in finding the right SB for you, do you ever wonder how you manage to attract the wrong kinds of sugar babies? or why it isn't working out for you?

Think: What do I have to offer? Is it what majority of sugar babies are looking for?

Location: Am I in a good location? Are there many SB's near me? Can I commute, or can they?

Profile: What does my profile represent? What am I putting out to the world?

Do not boast about holidays and money if that is not what you are prepared to give. Be honest with yourself as well as your SB.

Expectations: Are they too high? Too low?

Personality: Are you friendly? Boring? Maybe you need to be more outgoing or find someone who can bring that out of you.

When you set up your profile, you have to be very careful about what to place there. The result of what you put on your profile is whom you will attract.

Here are some examples:

If your profile is a blank canvas, then no SB will be messaging you or a very small amount will approach you. You have to try to make an effort if you would like someone to be attracted to you.

If you still decide that you'd rather have a blank profile, then you need to make up for it by not only introducing yourself in a spectacular way when sending a message, but also by sharing what you are like as a person, why you are on the website, what you hope to find and what you have to offer.

If you talk a lot about the money in your profile, especially as something that you have to offer, and even previous sugar babies that you had before. You are likely to attract two kinds of SBs. First are the SB who would like a PPM arrangement, the 'pro' who has more than one SD/SM; or you may attract more genuine SB, but it is highly unlikely. If PPM is what you are seeking then this will be a good way to go about it.

If you speak more about any of the following: holidays, gifts, hobbies, your profession, opportunities for the SB and/or a little bit about money, then you are likely to attract someone who would like to get into a SD/SM/SB arrangement. This may be long or short term depending on what you agree upon. This is likely to benefit you more as you can see them a few times a month and enjoy one another's company after coming to an agreement that suits you both.

You can speak about your life a little -- experiences that made you join the site, a little about money, travelling, hobbies, date ideas, maybe the number of children you have, your current situation If you are looking for something a little more serious, then you are likely to form a serious relationship with additional fun benefits. You can find a wonderful man or woman who you get to spoil and look after and who will also do the same for you, whilst living an amazing life together, full of different adventures. (exactly what my boyfriend and I have and it is the best!). It is simply two people in love, taking care of one another.

Now I know some of you do join to still find a very "normal" relationship with no money involved, no holidays planned, but just simply a good old pub with some company. Express that, do not hold back. There are women on these sites looking for the same exact thing you are. These women will usually be middle-aged women just looking for nice company and someone to love. They could even be young men or women simply looking to date someone older and wiser.

Assuming you have now found whom you were seeking.

How do you keep your SB interested? That's right, even with all the money or offers in the world, your SB can still become bored of you!

It is important to consider that this will not apply to those in a PPM or short-term SD/SM/SB arrangement. This goes for those who are in relationships or long-term arrangements.

You will need to engage well with your SB, make your presence known and have character. Being boring will leave nothing but a sour taste in their mouth. Seeing them as often as you can, random gift ideas, calling them and texting them just to let them know that they are on your mind are all simple ways of just keeping that connection alive and well. What happens when you can't hear someone on the phone? The connection fails or someone hangs up. Well you don't want the same thing to happen to your relationship because you are going M.I.A. Your other half will eventually fed up of trying to pursue you. Make sure you are present in their life even more so it's fine even if you aren't able to see each other as often as you'd like. It is also necessary to keep each other happy. I understand that getting comfortable is a great thing but getting comfortable enough to drop the ball and to make less effort is a definite no-no. Both of you need to make sure that you are still holding up your end to make the other person happy. All relationships and even arrangements require effort.

Another key element of this chapter is to not waste the SB's time or your own. It doesn't take a rocket scientist to work out that you'll start off by talking and getting to know several people but you have got to keep it real with them. Letting them know where you stand. Staying honest is vital. Do not lead them on if you have no real or good intentions with them. This especially goes for the SD/SM's who live abroad. If you have no intention of flying out the SB you are talking to then do not waste their time. Somebody out there will be willing to do what you are not. If you decide to meet, make reservations and stick to the dates. Do not cancel unless there's a death and do not turn up late. It does not take weeks to realise that you are not compatible. Most people work that out in the first few conversations. Do not lie about what you can provide. Do not give false hope and security. Stay true to yourself and stay true to them. Only come to an agreement that suits both of you.

The best advice I can give here is to stay true to yourself and it won't land you in any problems.

7: Discretion

This chapter concerns all because it is actually a thing where quite a few people go wrong and one of the reasons why relationships thrive. What is it you ask? DISCRETION PEOPLE! It pays to be discreet for several reasons and I'm going to get into them right this second.

The first reason is that putting all your business out to the world is never truly beneficial. You may say "but you had an article written about you" or "but you have written a book". Yes, to both BUT I know the difference between keeping the necessary and sacred things private and hiding your partner. I share very little about my life in general let alone share things about the person I love with the world. I never hide him, I simply protect our space and once you find someone that you cherish, you'll want to and should do the exact same. Maybe once we are married, I'll post a few wedding shots LOL. You do not have to be as private as my boyfriend and I are. Feel free to post a few pictures of yourselves here and there but never feel like you need to give the world an update anytime the two of you are up to anything.

In my case, I do not mention anything identifying about my boyfriend. I give up nothing too serious away about our relationship and best of all is that I keep him off social media. Now it's not because I'm ashamed of my boyfriend, it is because there are haters, jealous, slimy and cunning people in this world just waiting and praying that something bad will happen or that your happiness and blessings will come to an end. **DO NOT ALLOW ANYONE TO BLOCK YOUR BLESSINGS!** When I am out in public with him, we do not hide or shy away. We are very comfortable with seen with each other. That is what a relationship involves. I just do not deem it necessary to post and plaster everything we do together. Some things are just best left private. It allows you to cherish the sacred moments the two of you share together and nobody can put their two cents in. You'll be living your best life and holding it close to you at the same time. Not everybody needs to know your business. Your partner will appreciate that too.

The second reason is that your partner may require discretion. This can be broken down into two parts.

The first being (this is aimed mainly at those in a PPM or SD/SM/SB arrangement) that your partner is likely to either have a respectable job or a high profile one. The last thing they'll want is for their personal life to be out to the world. This goes both ways but applies mainly to SD/SMs. All they may want is to have a nice discreet lunch or some quiet fun with you without having to see it on the six o'clock news in the evening. Respect their wishes if they require discretion.

The second part is that rather than wanting discretion, they may **need** it. Keep in mind that your partner may be married or involved. They may have a job that they could lose if they were now in the public eye. Be respectful and simply enjoy your time together. If these circumstances change, roll with it.

Move in silence but you don't need to tip-toe. Just enjoy your life without having to prove anything to anyone.

8: Personal

I thought I'd take a little break from giving advice to talk about my boyfriend and I a little. However, not too much. It is just so you have a better understanding of how I am where I am today.

I also sensed that some may want to know a little about my boyfriend and I, and how it all came to be.

To clarify, I refer to my man as my boyfriend, **NOT** my sugar daddy. We just happened to meet on a sugar dating website. We are in a committed relationship and he keeps me completely happy the same way I keep him happy.

My boyfriend and I met online about a year ago and had a very honest conversation about our expectations from the beginning, even before we commence our relationship and I'm glad that we did because it has paid off for the both of us. There are no hidden agendas; everything is put on the table and is clear-cut. He is a man of principle and I try my best to be too. Things work out when the truth is told. We have stayed honest with each other for the duration of our relationship and it will continue to be that way. We know where the both of us stand in our relationship and we communicate in a healthy manner even on the bad days when we're both in our most vulnerable state, we pick each other back up, make up quick and get back to having fun. We know we would love to stay together and we both know what we each have to do to ensure that happens. Effective communication is vital when it comes to maintaining the special bond you share. Had he lied, led me on and just wasted my time, it would not have worked out but we both made things crystal clear to each other and set a date to meet almost immediately to avoid any doubt and cause for concern. Now, my boyfriend lives abroad so he booked his flight to come and see me we then got to know each other on an amazing first date in Chelsea, London, and the rest is history! We have had nothing but good times. Because he lives abroad, he often purchases my tickets to go and see him, we have an amazing time together; we go to amazing restaurants and bars or he will book his ticket to London and we do the same here. He lacks nothing in the gentleman department as he showers me with amazing holidays throughout the year with more coming up and also gifts. They vary from a few Chanel bags to designer shoes and helps me out financially when I need it. Not to mention, he is the reason I have been able to publish my book by supporting my every move, believing in my potential, trusting that I know what I am doing and funding the release! So, it is all thanks to God, my boyfriend and my mother for raising an amazing daughter that I am able to share these gems with you.

For all of whom are still thinking that 'if he had no money then she'd leave', or 'if she didn't look good or spread her legs then he'd leave', you still have a lot to learn so keep reading. That could not be further from the truth. Those aspects do play a role in the relationship, yes, but that is not the sole reason why we are together. Our love for each other runs deeper than that. Much deeper.

Ladies, get a man who'll scoop up your sick with his bare

hands when you clog the drain and put your drunk self to bed (this happened on or around our fourth date so pretty early on). We were both by this time completely infatuated with one another, I'm good woman to him too, and don't you forget it. That's the love I have in my life and wouldn't dream of losing it so why wouldn't I be a good woman to him? We both deserve the best. Gross, but cute, right? First and last time he'll have to do that!

The point was, I was in a very bad state and he took care of me. It goes beyond just 'having a good time'. I'd give my life for this man.

He is also a great mentor, an amazing support system and a highly intelligent man. It astonishes me! It helps that we are both fluent in French and he speaks several other languages. Holidays are never a struggle that way. Best of all, he loves me with all his heart and I wouldn't have it any other way.

I love him too and honey, for when you read this, this is my written public display of affection and gratitude. You are amazing!

Don't you worry guys, I enrich his life in many different ways myself. He is a man of very few words but he shows me often that he loves me, appreciates me, and acknowledge what I do for him and happiness that I bring into his life. It is how we complement one another. I just thought it would be slightly strange, maybe even a little cocky to brag about how I make someone happy (I'll leave that to him) so I just took this opportunity to gush about my man, show him some more appreciation and write about how he has changed my life for the better.

9: Opportunities

This chapter is for all the SB's out there. I'd like for you to really take this one in. The phrase 'seize your opportunities' fits perfectly here. GUYS! GIRLS! Do **NOT** limit your options to simply receiving money and going on holiday. You're dating someone with status and you're just going to be in the same spot you were in before you met him? No. Level up! Always level up. Allow them to motivate you into being the best version of yourself and reach your potential because you can. The person you are with has not gotten to where they are today without making some important friends along the way. See what job/career doors he or she can open up for you. Better yet, maybe they can invest in your start up business or help you to promote and improve certain aspects. There is so much that your SD/SM can do for you if you are open to those possibilities. Your SD/SM will want nothing more than for you to do better in life and for yourself too. Another smart idea would be to invest some of the money they give to you into a project or idea you have. Maybe even save it for a rainy day. You can't be completely poor but wearing the latest designer items. It doesn't make sense and it isn't an attractive trait to constantly need money.

Your SD/SM will offer it, sure. But to always need something from them every day will show them that you are just leeching off of them and making no real effort or progress in your life (this goes for those who are already receiving a lot of money as part of the agreement yet still need more).

TIP: if you have those designer items and you still need money but you feel as though you'll be pushing it by asking for more money, sell the item. Tell your partner the situation and sell it. They'd rather you have money than be poor. Just make sure that the designer items that you do buy or receive as a gift, hold their value or appreciate in value (why I pick Chanel bags) otherwise you'll be losing out.

Asking for money however to invest is a different story and could actually impress them. If you are dating someone influential then use it to your advantage! They'll be happy to help. Present your business ideas, mood board, and 5-year plan and take it from there. Show them that you are serious about it before asking for a penny. This way they will understand just how serious you are.

10: Unconventional Relationships

Throughout this book, we have covered PPM, SD/SM/SB arrangements, relationships with additional benefits and the more conventional relationship as the main types of relationships.

In the sugaring world, there any many more options for you to choose from or potentially be offered.

People on dating sites are looking for all sorts of different things, such as:

Being in a cuckold relationship/arrangement: this scenario is mainly an SD that would like to meet an SB who is happy to have sexual relations with other men. The degree of how far those sexual encounters needs to clear in advance between the two of you. The SD may even be dominating, he would find it appealing that the men the SB is having a physical relationship with know about him. He may even pay the SB to do this for his benefit or for the man involved. He may find a place for this all to happen or pay for the location being used.

Joining a couple in their relationship: this could be a married couple, or a boyfriend and girlfriend looking to add a third member to their relationship. The SB may be given an allowance for being part of their relationship. The SB may be given duties, and may receive a job offer. Usually the SB would need to be bisexual in nature for this arrangement to work. There is a high chance the SB will be sexually involved with the already established couple.

Having a SD/SB with multiple SB's: ah, the playboy life. The SD/SB may not want to have just one SB so the SB would be required to be okay with that. You will more than likely be taken care of financially. The SD/SM will almost certainly be dominant in nature so if you are quite combative, this is not for you. If you are not bisexual, this may also not be for you. This offer however, could bring to you great career opportunities. The kind of SD/SM's that prefer this arrangement also love to see their SB's thrive!

Being the dominator to a slave: here the SB will dominate the SD/SM. They may cross-dress for you. They may give you money to be able to be themselves around you. You'll sexually and potentially financially dominate them. They will be willing to do household chores for you. The SB will be the boss. Whatever the SB says, goes.

Being the slave to the dominator: the SB will be the slave in this situation. They will have to adhere to what the SD/SM is ordering. The domination is usually put into action in the bedroom though some like to be dominant constantly. The SB may have to call the SD/SM a certain name and follow a few rules. BDSM is highly likely to be a factor. Being open-minded and kinky would definitely go a long way for this arrangement. While the SD/SM is going to take care of your needs, this will not be the priority nor the focus of this agreement so keep that in mind.

Working for an SD/SB and having sexual relations: think of this as sleeping with the boss because, well... essentially that is what it is. You will be employed by the SD/SM and will be involved with them as well. It is unlikely that this will be a relationship but a fantasy of sorts. The SB may be a cleaner or personal assistant. Depending on who the SD/SM is, you may even get to travel around the world with them whilst they fund your stay. The SB will be getting a salary and if the SB is pleasing them in many ways, maybe with even something extra.

Online arrangement: this might be one of the least popular types of arrangements because well, pornography exists. BUT you still have a few SD/SM's who like to pay for something exclusive and something that only they are seeing. This arrangement is usually long distance and takes place every so often. The SD/SM may not give you money but the two of you may just exchange whatever you decide online. The two of you could even become pen pals. Just be sure to know whom it is you are talking to behind or on the other end.

I hope that you have become more aware of what can happen in the dating world and the sugaring world. It can be rather overwhelming but everybody's thinking about joining, has already joined and that has already found someone will be just fine. You will all find your way. I have been exactly where you are with that 'lost' feeling and now here I am, I have found myself, I have found myself a nice man and I have found myself in your mind where you are registering the advice I am giving so you can do the exact same.

11: Gold Digger vs. Sugar Baby

In this paragraph, I'd like to explain the difference between a '**gold digger**' and a '**sugar baby**'. Though many people may think that they are the same, I can tell you that there are many differences between the two! Anything from the manner in which one may lead their life, to what they may expect from the person that they are with. How a person treats you is also an indication of whether they are a gold digger or a sugar baby.

There is a big stigma when it comes to sugar dating and this is mainly because it is common to put both titles in the same boat. So, I will shed some light on the main differences and what we should ALL look out for.

The term gold digger has been used from the 1900s with records even dating back as far as the 1830s. A gold digger is usually in the form of a young woman (though not limited to) and will date or marry a man (or woman) purely for material and financial gains and benefits. She or he will have no intention of forming a genuine connection with the said person, but will stay in the relationship for their individual purpose.

Now, I have to clarify something else in this paragraph, which is that not all gold diggers are female. That's right ladies! Hold on tight to your purses because male gold diggers are around too! Not all are young, some are even middle-aged or elders. Many are pros and in the form of con artists. They may appear to be in a certain way but it couldn't be farther from the truth.

How to distinguish whether you are dating a gold digger or a sugar baby you ask? Wait no more because I have all the answers right here.

Aims/goals for a gold digger:

- Will use you to climb the social or business ladder: Now, there is nothing wrong with introducing your partner to some very important people or presenting them with amazing opportunities, BUT do they seem more interested in the people and opportunities than you do? **There is your red flag.**
- Money, money, money. What else? All they will talk about is money; they will always have a need for it. They will talk about needing and wanting money so much that you will hear that echo in your sleep. It will be never-ending. You will be spending more on them than you have spent in your lifetime! **Be careful!**

Character traits for a gold digger:

- Money oriented – a gold digger will be around when there is money to spend on him or her but gone without a second thought when the money dries up or there is a pause in the spending. You will see a yo-yo effect with a gold digger, close to you when you have money to spend on them, couldn't be further away from you, maybe even ending contact with you when you have not got a certain amount of money to spend. They will be gone the second no money is offered. Pity. They will only love the money, they won't love you.

- No goals or ambition – though money might not be the only thing you have to offer, it certainly is the only thing a gold digger will be interested in. They won't hold jobs down for very long, not studying, aren't concerned about being unemployed, will solely rely on the money you are providing. If you present them with some great opportunity, they will sabotage it by not taking it seriously or not working hard enough. They will have no drive, behave as though the world owes them something and it will be apparent from the start. They would rather have expensive items instead of keeping their bills paid for. They do not prioritise and seem a little lost. **Stay away!**
- Selfish and lazy – they will make no efforts towards you. They will take no interest in getting to know you as a person or building a serious relationship or at least a solid foundation/bond between the two of you. It will be all about them, so do not be surprised if they cannot even spell your surname! They will constantly take from you and never give. **It is a dangerous position to be in.**

I'll elaborate a little more in two sections.

<u>Signs that **SHE** is a gold digger:</u>

1. She **ONLY** wants expensive gifts. We all love expensive gifts (myself included) but if getting her something sentimental or cheaper will make her foam at the mouth with rage then run for your life. If she gets angry or becomes aloof, she's playing you and you are playing yourself.

2. She is a bit too curious about your financial status. She will want to know the ins and outs of what you are paid for, and how much it pays. She should take an interest in your work of course and the question could casually come up but her interest should not be focused on what your annual income is looking like. You should disclose that when you are ready to. She'll take things at face value – the car you drive, the house you live in, etc. You have been warned! Not all that glitters is gold. A man could live in a palace and be declared bankrupt. Another man could live in a small apartment and be making a fortune! Do not judge a man by what he chooses to initially show you, there could be more to him – good AND bad.

<u>NOTE TO WOMEN:</u> A RICH MAN CAN HAVE £100,000,00 AND GIVE YOU £100. A POOR MAN CAN HAVE £100 AND GIVE YOU £90. Do not judge a book by its cover.

3. She **NEVER** pays. Never offers even a small sentimental gift, doesn't treat you on your birthday,

doesn't get you something just because she thinks you'd like it. Doesn't get you anything as a sign of appreciation for everything you have done for her. Takes what you do for her for granted. Shows no gratitude.

4. Hates other women. This depends a lot on the scenario. Most women will only show signs of disapproval towards women that have shown signs of flirtatiousness or if their man has been the one doing the flirting. In this case, it is acceptable to voice that. But, in a gold diggers case, she will become insecure around any women at all as she doesn't want to lose any of the privileges she is being showered with. She will view another woman as a threat when there is no sign of the other woman and man flirting or getting close. This includes strangers. She will loathe female company around the man she is dating. If your partner has given you no reason to doubt their loyalty, then do not doubt their loyalty.

   <u>NOTE TO MEN:</u> THIS DOES NOT MEAN YOU SHOULD GO OUT OF YOUR WAY TO MAKE HER FEEL INSECURE. ALWAYS REASSURE YOUR LADY, ESPECIALLY AROUND OTHER WOMEN!

5. She uses her looks for short-term gains. She will use sex appeal to get anything she may need from everyone. There is nothing wrong with using sex appeal with your partner. Heck, it is one of our advantages as women! In saying that, if she does this with everyone, that is where the problem lies. Anyone she sees as useful will be seeing her exposed cleavage.

6. Obsessed with status. She will want the man that she's with to hold an important position in society. If he isn't well known or she considers him to be a nobody (even if he is wealthy) she will disappear in a second.
7. The sense of entitlement. No long-term goals. She needs to live an extravagant lifestyle constantly and believes that she deserves it. She will talk about what she has done and worn with arrogance.

Signs that **HE** is a gold digger:

1. Always has financial emergencies. Borrows money from you, promises to pay you back but never does. Always has to help a certain friend you have never heard of or seen.
2. More interested in your finances. He will constantly talk about your finances constantly rather than spend quality time with you. Some men are worse than women, when it comes to this! He will ask you to invest your money in some questionable business schemes but never involve you in them or keep you in the loop! You will not profit from this investment.
3. No clear ambition. Most gold diggers are not ambitious. They have no plan to do anything with themselves apart from spending your money.
4. Unemployed or lies about his job.
5. Views you as his ATM machine. He knows your paydays. Whenever you give him some money, there is no "thank you". He sees you as a walking currency sign.

The term 'sugar daddy' can be traced as far back as the 1920s. This later led to the term 'sugar baby', which stemmed from the popularity of candy in the 1930s. Sugar baby is used to describing women for the most part (though it doesn't exclude men) who date (mostly older) men (or women) who can improve and be a positive influence in their lives in more ways than just one. Over the years, the term has taken on new meanings as people have adapted to sugar dating.

People have come up with new concepts and use sugar dating to open those doors. There are endless possibilities when it comes to sugar dating. Whatever you look for in a partner, be sure that someone else is also looking for the same thing and dating on sugar dating sites make it just that much easier to find.

Character traits for a sugar baby:

- Has goals and is passionate about them. She or he is driven to succeed and will make the most of the opportunities presented to them. They will stop at nothing to make something out of their lives and will work very hard to get to where they need to be. They will encourage their sugar daddy or sugar mummy to help, mentor, guide, and possibly finance after presenting detailed information about the business venture, and will always keep their SD/SM updated. The SD/SM may even be a willing partner in this venture or could just be happy that their SB is doing well for themselves.

- Always perseveres to reach her goals. Never gives up and always strives to be the best and for the best. Shows great courage.

- A SB is honest with her partner and has no complex. They will state what they'd like without pretending they're not interested in what you have to offer. A SB doesn't fear your reaction as they would rather be upfront about everything instead of being misleading. You will not be going in blind, as you'll know what you are in for. You can also be just as honest with them. The two of you will come to a mutual understanding of what will make the pair of you happy.

- They give and take. It is common to gift and treat your SB and they will be happy receiving these luxurious treats but a SB will also give. It may not be as expensive as anything you have ever given them but it is the thought that counts. They're working with what they've got. I mean, what do you get a man or woman that already has everything? His/her dream man/woman will most likely get them something sentimental and it'll mean the world to the SD/SM. It may even cost a pretty penny too. SBs' never be afraid or against gifting your partner. They'll always be happy to do it for you when they know you really appreciate them.

- Classy, not trashy. Will certainly dress to impress and have the personality to match. Someone you will not only look at but also listen to them as they send you into a deep trance. You will get lost in their eyes and voice and think you are a very blessed person. That is the type of sugar baby that you need.
Female SBs: they will walk and the whole room will be thinking how did he/she get her? She is stunning! When you talk to her, she will also have substance and character. Someone who will keep you on your toes. Oh, and someone who also knows how to use their cutlery correctly.

- Humble. A humble SB will remember their beginnings and will not get too big headed. They will show no signs of arrogance but instead are eager to learn more about life. They are happy to keep exploring and having fun whilst being spoiled and doing some spoiling themselves. It isn't all about them but it is about the two of you together.

- Interested. A SB will show the utmost respect and interest to their SD/SM. They will regularly check up on him/her. Ensure that their partner is okay and just keep the spark going, the good vibes will be consistent and should there be a hiccup in the arrangement/relationship, they won't let that stop them from caring for their SD/SM and will make the relationship or arrangement work. They certainly won't be willing to give up on their partner because of minor issues (in some cases major) and will encourage their partner to do the same. They are open to more than just an arrangement which means they see a future with that person. A SB is not flaky and will certainly stick around. If a SB is your girlfriend then she will be in it for the long run.

12: Dating in the Real World

There are some of you reading this book who prefer to get out there and actively get involved in the dating world. Don't worry, I got you guys covered too. Just think of me as a guru at this point.

Let's start with the gentlemen first. I feel as though you may have it slightly harder than women do, to confront dating in real life head on. I'm here to help. It is easy to be taken as arrogant or sleazy, maybe even cocky when approaching a lady or a man when you are only trying to show how confident you are. Honestly, the best thing to do here, is have a swig of your drink, take a deep breath and just go over to show her/him the sweet gentleman that you are. There is no need to put on an act. Women/men will see right through it and it is at that point that the situation will backfire. Just be yourself. If you have bad jokes, tell them. If you have something interesting to talk about, say it! I am telling you if he/she doesn't go for it then guess what? You are simply not compatible. That doesn't mean that there is anything wrong with you. It simply wasn't meant to be.

What if you feel like a fool because the woman says she has a boyfriend? Or says that she is a lesbian or cuddles up to her best friend to pretend to be one? Well, back away. Do not be a douche and still try to work your way in. That is the female's indirect way of telling you, she has no interest in getting to know you.

Where to go? Well, this one would depend on where you

are geographically so I have to generalise a little here. If you live in London, the obvious place to go in central London or its surrounding areas! Oxford Street, Charing cross, Embankment, Covent Garden, Leicester Square, Mayfair, Liverpool Street, Cannon street, Paddington, Piccadilly, Soho, Marylebone, Chelsea, Battersea and many more! There are great restaurants, bars, clubs, even pubs to meet amazing women/men. These are also amazing areas where you can go on a date. Everything around you just comes to light and the atmosphere is so great!

Wear something smart and casual. I had mentioned the crisp white shirt earlier in the book because it works like a charm. Pastel colours are a pretty good look too. Vraiment chic pour les homme. A nice pair of smart looking jeans or chinos will work. Maybe even throw on a jacket/blazer with some moccasins on your feet and you sir, are good to go!

If you are from **out of London** then please feel free to divert your attention to the **midsection** of the **ladies' paragraph below**.

Ladies!

What is there to say really? We have it easier than the men do. Simply because we are not expected to make the first move to get your beautiful ass in gear, move it and make the most of what your mama gave you! You will not find your future man by living the life of a hermit. Live the life of Riley instead! Doll yourselves up, put that pretty dress or skirt on with those sexy heels (flats or socks in your bag ladies), do your hair and makeup and get out there with your girls to socialise!

Go to the bar, bat your eyelashes, give that sultry look and smile, and allow your personality to do the rest. If you are brave enough, you can make the first move! After a few cocktails, we have the confidence of a stuntman so put it to good use. Get some numbers, and get talking to people. I'll give you the same advice as I gave the men, go up into London if you are anywhere around there.

Since I focused on London locations in the gentleman's section, I'll focus on the out of London areas here. If you are from **London** then feel free to read the **midsection** of the **gentleman's paragraph above**.

There are still lovely and beautiful places to go no matter where you live! Go to your local city centre. There are likely to be nice, and local bars and restaurants where you can meet some people and enjoy a good laugh. If you live in the middle of nowhere then I suggest you commute to where there is a sign of human life rather than cattle.

Since there may not be many places to go to, dressed up and eat/drink in, maybe there are a few dance classes or social events you can attend. Social events such as weddings and sports events are a great way of meeting people, potentially your partner. A great way to network, flirt and socialise.

It is more than possible to meet someone in the real world but these things take time. It also means you'd need to dedicate your precious time and energy into going out (and spending money) often. This is the reason why most people date online initially until they feel as though they are speaking to someone who is worth meeting and worth taking out on a date to get to know them. However, for those of you who still like to literally actively date and get out there, I hope that this has been a rather enlightening chapter for you.

13: Sugar Dating Countries

This section of my book is not a particularly lengthy one. It is rather informative. However, it is important to work with your logistics. If you are open to trying out the sugar dating way then it is good to know whether it is something that is possible near where you live.

I have put together some countries and even cities so you may have a clearer understanding about where sugar dating is most popular and where you can easily 'bag' yourself a sugar daddy, sugar mummy or sugar baby!

In this age, the dating game is getting really hard. People are now more aware of what they want and because of dating websites and apps, it's easy for them to get into sugar dating. Modern countries where sugar dating is most widely acknowledged and most active are Australia, the United Kingdom, the United States of America, and Canada. These countries all have a booming economy, a rich culture, and an interest in individual freedom, which supports sugar dating.

North America.

When it comes to dating a sugar daddy, the most difficult part may be in finding them.

Based on where you live, the number of sugar daddies, who are available, might not be sufficient for them to simply be found. It is because every community is different as well as every country. Of course, there are 10 cities in the U.S., in particular, that stand out from amongst the rest.

Consider how much easier your life would be if you find a true connection and achieve your career goals. You can do what you really wanted to, go on vacation, treat yourself to massages and enjoy lavish dinners.

Are you with me?

Here's the thing: That lifestyle is possible.

You just need to find a sugar daddy or a wealthy boyfriend who is happy to do the same.

It's quite unsurprising that with a population as huge and diverse as America, that it has a market for the sugar dating culture. Sugar daddies – the approved name granted to those wealthy men – and the microcosm they inhabit isn't anything new. They emerged as a group during America's student-debt crises.

The year 2014 saw a huge spike in sugar dating nationwide, particularly in southern states.

Some of the states show higher rates of sugar relationships

than others as the views and acceptability of this type of dating is based on location. Sugar babies often use their extra income to pay off their college fees, rent and credit card bills. Popular dating websites now make it easy for men and women looking for a new sugar daddy, sugar baby or sugar mummy to be picky of their choosing and to find someone who they can trust and be happy with. Sugar daddies in America are generous to all the beautiful and sexy sugar babies. I have prepared the list of top 10 cities in America along with statistic where sugar dating is most popular:

1. Atlanta (5.98 sugar daddies per 1000 men)
2. Scottsdale (5.23 sugar daddies per 1000 men)
3. San Francisco (4.94 sugar daddies per 1000 men)
4. Tampa (4.48 sugar daddies per 1000 men)
5. Boston (4.29 sugar daddies per 1000 men)
6. Las Vegas (4.17 sugar daddies per 1000 men)
7. Orlando (3.98 sugar daddies per 1000 men)
8. Log Angeles (3.61 sugar daddies per 1000 men)
9. Seattle (3.47 sugar daddies per 1000 men)
10. Austin (3.13 sugar daddies per 1000 men)

This may sound like there are barely any sugar daddies around but keep in mind that these figures aren't the most recent and they have considerably risen over the last few years! I'd go as far as saying, it'd be very hard not to find a sugar daddy for yourself in the United States.

During 2007, the figures for married sugar daddies have

fallen from **46% to 33%.** This goes to show that the sugar world is getting more acknowledged among single men. An average U.S. sugar daddy is **42** years old with an average income of **$524,127.** They spend an average of **$5,693** per month on sugar babies. The University of Texas at Austin, in specific, saw a huge growth in sign-ups between 2013 and 2014.

Now all this data reveals that not only is this phenomenon spreading, but it's also gaining traction in a number of more areas.

Consider the Following before You Meet Your Sugar Baby, Sugar Daddy or Sugar Mummy in America:

What time of the day will you meet up, and for how many hours?
The exact place where will you meet (it could be a hotel, sugar baby's place or sugar daddies/mummies home)?
What will a usual date involve (theatre, lunch, travel, long walks, cocktail events, movies)?
Will you hang out on your own, or will you be seen in public together?
When will you get rewards/payment/gifts/etc.?
How long do you expect this relationship to last?
What does each of you reflect a deal breaker (failed to make on-time payments, the last-minute termination, the finding that you're not completely dating each other, or a demand is thought too greedy)?

<u>Sugar Dating Rules in the U.S.</u>

- ✓ Oblige to identity online and IRL
- ✓ Do your work, and be tolerant
- ✓ Be upfront
- ✓ Sketch a specific, equally beneficial agreement
- ✓ Never get too easy
- ✓ Stick to the agreement
- ✓ Be discrete
- ✓ Maximise the relationship
- ✓ Manage your prospects
- ✓ Have a Plan-B

<u>London</u>

There is plenty of wealthy men/woman in the UK. It is also considered as the most advanced country. Sugar daddies and mummies in London are pursuing some sexy babies to spoil. They have reached a certain status in their professions and are using online dating sites to find potential sugar babies to spend their money on and even possibly grow very fond of. Sugar babies, on the other hand, need wealthy sugar daddies/mummies to support them. What's more, they need sugar daddies/mummies to give them a chance to support their career plans and ventures. It doesn't just stop there; some arrangements even end up turning into relationships or they may even start off that way!

Whether it's because of high salaries in cities in the UK,

such as London, or the appalling weather which leaves the UK population with little to do on vacation, there is no lack of women or men pursuing sugar daddies/mummies in London. The job market is hard and with growing debts from the ever-increasing university fees, young women/men here are on the look-out for someone to show them a different and better side to life and treat them to things that they cannot afford. See the list I have made for the top 10 cities in the UK, where sugar dating is prevalent.

1. London
2. Birmingham
3. Edinburgh
4. Liverpool
5. Manchester
6. Bristol
7. Glasgow
8. Leeds
9. Cardiff
10. Nottingham

Higher fee costs and accommodation in London are making students look for new ways to earn some cash while studying. In the UK precisely, around 160,000 which make up 40% of the 400,000 individuals on dating sites are student sugar babies, a figure which most of the sites claimed go off in 2012 when universities started charging up to £9,000 in fees per year. During 2017, around 75,000 UK students registered with sugar daddy websites. For some, sugar daddies/mummies are less of a necessity and more a means to enjoy a better lifestyle, allowing them to travel, party, and live in better accommodation and even fall in love. With the help of a sugar daddy or mummy, they can travel to different cities, shop on regular basis, eat out in the city and more. There are also sugar baby summits held in London where both sugar babies come together. Keep an eye out. The summits are usually all about sugar babies coming together to learn how to maximise their sugar experience. There are also some meet and greets between sugar babies and sugar daddies that are also held all over the world.

Besides London, another popular city for finding a sugar daddy is **Leeds.** The acceptance here has grown quite a bit amongst men who were working in London and moved here for a quiet lifestyle. With numerous exclusive clubs, bars, and restaurants, there is an abundant place for a sugar baby to meet his/her perfect man.

In **Edinburgh**, sugar babies can find sugar daddies/mummies who are not just financially stable but also emotionally prepared to start this kind of relationship. In Edinburgh, men are known to be more sensitive so if you are seeking an emotional connection, this is the right place for meeting that kind of a man.

Manchester is another potential city for finding sugar daddies. Numerous aspiring men and women live here who have capitalised on stocks and businesses which have made them handsome money. They want to share it with beautiful and sexy sugar babies out there.

<u>Note:</u> All of these locations are prime spots for women and men to find the right sugar relationship. As long as you are upfront about your expectations, you will not be let down!

14: Dating 101

This section of the book was a spur of the moment afterthought. I figured, no matter how much I explain what to do throughout the book, life has a funny way of throwing us curveballs. It is hard to predict what to do in what type of situation. I've decided to put together a few FAQs and different kinds of common scenarios and advise what to do and the best outcome. This will also include some dating 101 tips.

Let's start with the FAQs:

Should I pay for a membership?

Read what the website has to offer, maybe some reviews. Look at the ratio between men and women. Join first, have a look around and make the decision about whether you like the look of some profiles. Alternatively, you can wait until someone sends you a message before upgrading your account. Most dating sites have free membership for women and/or men.

I've been on a site for a long time with no success, I feel like giving up. What do I do?

Be patient. Not everyone can meet their future partner overnight. These things can take time. It will be worth the wait once the person you are meant to date comes

along. You'll find that the right person will come when you least expect it. Just let your guards down.

We have been talking perfectly fine one day and the next they disappear/become strange. What have I done wrong? What should I do now?

Remember this: as you begin to date, the both of you will be talking to several other people and getting to know them. They will decide to continue to interact with the person they feel most connected to and it might not be you. This also applies to the other party, you may decide to continue your journey with one person in particular and stop talking to the two or three other people. It isn't anything personal, it is all about chemistry. Do not think that you have done anything wrong if you have been ghosted. Just pick yourself up and check out your other options.

We've met but it seems we are no longer on the same page. How do I change their mind?

You can't. If the two of you are on different pages then the vibes will be off. Do not force it. Wish each other well and move on.

I only get approached by someone who wants something completely different than I do. How do I attract the right people?

It's simple really, you reap what you sow. You get what you put out. Be true to yourself, you'll receive someone genuine who is on the same page. Do not settle for less than what you deserve.

How long did it take you to find your boyfriend?

It took me a couple of weeks if that. We were fortunate enough to meet each other quickly after joining the site.

How do you make it work?

Communication is key. As long as there is effective communication between the two of you. Things should go smoothly.

How do I get nice things from my partner?

Be a good partner. If the 'nice things' were on the table before the two of you got together then he/she will be happy to treat you as long as you are nothing but good to them.

Scenarios:

Conversations are going well, but all of a sudden, they disappear. What to do?

Accept it. If you chase it any more then it'll be a waste of your own time. They may even ignore you if you keep sending them messages. You are entitled to send a 'closure' message to make sure things really are over between the two of you.

You are talking, but he/she lives abroad. They're meant to pay for your ticket to fly over so the two of you can meet but it's been a while and no real progress. What to do?

If he/she wants to book your ticket they will. If the two of you agree on a date, the next step is to book tickets. Whether it is you to fly over or them to fly to you. If the tickets aren't booked within a couple of weeks of talking about it and agreeing on a date, move on.

My date cancelled last minute. What do I do?

Think! What was the reason they had to cancel? Is it an acceptable reason or is it a pitiful excuse? How many times have they cancelled? Is it the first or third time? How long before you have planned to meet have they cancelled? One day or one hour before? How much do you actually like them? Not enough to move on? Not enough to deal with the wasted time?

The person I'm talking to doesn't want to talk on the phone/keeps stalling/send a picture.

They're wasting your time. Do not pursue this.

The date was a waste of time. What should I do?

It's a shame for that to happen but sometimes it does. Express that it was nice meeting them but it will not work out for a said reason and then move on.

I think I have found someone suited to me but they live out of town. What do I do?

It helps to drive or have a licence so you can hire a car. It helps if your partner is ready and willing to drive if you cannot or pay for your car journey. If it is a few hours away, coach or train is your best bet.

I'm in a PPM/sugar baby and sugar daddy or mum arrangement. I met with him/her but it is nothing like we had discussed it would be. Are they stalling to start the arrangement?

If you feel like your date wants to get their end of the arrangement sorted but not cater to yours then do not go for it. Make sure the both of you know how it is going to work before the meeting.

I've been speaking to a SD/SB/SM for a few weeks but the conversation has now died down and we no longer communicate. What should I do?

Either set an ultimatum and insist on meeting very soon or leave it alone and move on.

I have been dating a SD/SM and we are on the same page but it is taking a long time for the arrangement to get off the ground.

Speak to the person you are dating about it. Be upfront and honest otherwise the situation will remain the same. Do not become pushy or make the person feel any type of pressure. Have an adult conversation without making yourself a burden to your date.

I have been dating a SD/SM but I don't think I'm their only SB.

Make sure the two of you are practising safe sex if you are okay with this situation. If not, tell your SD/SM and see what they say. Make an informed decision based on how you feel as a result of their response.

My SD/SM/SB is into some really weird things (in/out of the bedroom). What should I do?

Does it make you feel uncomfortable or are you open to trying them? This is a conversation you should have with

each other before reaching the stage where it comes into practice. The two of you should feel safe and secure in each other's presence.

Should I send money before I meet someone?

The short answer is no. it is vital to meet the person you are willing to financially assist. If your arrangement is strictly online and money needs to be sent then make sure to audio or face call someone before doing so.

How do I tell who is fake and who is genuine?

Most people will prove their real intentions from the very beginning. Remember that if the person is serious about dating you, they will make it work no matter what. If they don't, then they are not the person for you.

How do I keep our meetings discreet?

Easy. Go to places neither of you will be recognised. If it isn't an issue for you then feel free to stay local to where you live. However, it is just good fun and a good experience to venture out.

How do I deal with rejection?

Rejection is never an easy thing to deal with. It is very

common in the dating world for everyone. There are many different reasons why someone may get rejected aside from their physical appearance. Things like goals, behaviour, personality etc. all come into question. Do not take it personally, it is a common occurrence and always a blessing in disguise. There is someone for everyone out there.

Dating 101:

It's always nice to go somewhere amazing with the upper-class socialites. A man may take you to somewhere a little below that. Do not be offended. Some men test character to see whether the lady/man that they are dating is shallow or not. Keep this in mind. No matter what the situation or what the two of you have agreed, it is always good to be comfortable and happy with who you are with no matter the environment. This mainly applies to those who are in a relationship, a serious/long-term sugar relationship, or dating with the intention of ending up in a relationship.

With that being said, by no means is it acceptable to be not be taken on a joy-ride. HOWEVER, remain humble at ALL costs. I'll tell you what I have told a good friend of mine, you both owe each other nothing at all and your partner will please you from the kindness of their heart.

SD's/SM's you need to be humble because boasting about your money, the number of people you've slept with, your in-depth experience with previous SB's will do nothing but turn your SB off. Take pride in what you have achieved in your life but do not allow arrogance to cloud the better part of your personality.

SB's you also need to remain extremely humble. The LAST thing you want anyone to say to you is "you wouldn't have this/be here if it wasn't for me". Do not act like your daddy is the King because he isn't. you need your SD/SM's help and remaining humble is the only way for them to see behind the façade. So, there is no need to act all high and mighty because they may just take you down a notch. Do not act like a bush person but also do not behave as though you have your life in complete order either.

Do not sweat the small stuff. If you fly economy, eat in a run-down restaurant or go through a poverty-stricken area. Do not make a fuss! There will be more positives than negatives! In fact, let the less fun experience be a topic of conversation for you and a growing curve! If you eat in a bad restaurant once, laugh about it and swear never to go back. You may fly economy and stay in a five-star hotel! Feed elephants, go to a breath-taking beach. You will block all those blessings if you get held up on the fact that you flew economy for several hours. That minor detail is so insignificant compared to the experience of a lifetime that is waiting for you on the other side It'll be something you end up being grateful for because you have experienced it together and I am sure your SD/SM will offer something more upgraded next time.

Know your list of non-negotiables. Try not to include

physical attributes. Do they smoke? Are they non-monogamous? Have they eternally dedicated Saturday nights to 'the guys'? Put this into perspective before wasting your time.

Do not prejudge your date. They may surprise you and be an even better person than you imagined.

Do not compare your new boyfriend/girlfriend or sugar daddy/mummy to any ex's or previous experiences. No two people are the same so be open-minded and accepting of new circumstances.

Be open to love. The case may be that some people have become emotionally unavailable. Well, your relationships won't work that way. No matter what type of relationship it is. Open your mind and heart. Allow yourself to love and be loved. You may get hurt but it important to form bonds and beautiful connections with people. It is how we grow and develop best.

Do not be afraid of treating and spoiling your partner. Men, I know many of you will be the one taking care of the bill and looking after your lady/man. In spite of that, ladies, do not allow the man/woman you are dating to feel as though their efforts are going unappreciated. Do something nice for them, a meaningful gift with a lot of sentiment. Your small gesture will go a long way.

Watch your alcohol intake. You do not want to be in a vulnerable state with someone you are not familiar with or leave a bad impression. This is important especially on the first date.

Do not block your own blessings by being too picky. We all have standards as I've previously mentioned but go for someone different! Maybe, someone, you wouldn't find attractive initially. Beauty is not just skin deep, it goes way beyond that. It could be the best thing to ever happened to you. You can't get better results if you repeat the same mistakes. Their personality, character traits may be everything you have ever hoped for and you may not get to see that all because you're caught up on their hair colour.

If you have a dating 'must have' list, get rid of it. There is more to life than someone's height and facial hair. They may be visually impressive but have the personality of a brick wall.

Be honest with yourself and with the person you're with. You should not expect the person you're with to have to read between the lines. It is best to air out what it is you expect from each other.

Try not to be a harsh critic when it comes to someone's performance in the bedroom. Tell them what you like and how you like it. Coach them. It'll get better from there. Set your boundaries and then go from there.

Have a positive outlook on life. Have good energy. Be pleasant to be around.

Be nice to those around you especially in the company of the person you are dating. No arrogance towards the waiters or criticism about someone's outfit. Unless of course, that is your thing. Then go right ahead! It'll be a bonding experience. Knock yourselves out – just keep your voices down.

Say please and thank you. if your date opens doors, pulls chairs out, orders your food. Show your gratitude. Do more than thank them verbally (if you know what I mean) if you really like/love them.

Pay attention to things that may raise concern. Red flags are often ignored but shouldn't be. Is there something he/she does that doesn't seem right? Do they withhold important information? Do they avoid and change subjects as soon as something comes up? Be aware. They are under no obligation to divulge private information but the basic 'get to know' questions should be answered.

Affection is important. Allow the person you are with to **FEEL** what you feel about them. Do not neglect that.

Call or text them! Do not wait just to seem 'cool'. You may come across as disinterested instead. It is good to show your interest. Just don't allow all the effort to be one-sided. It is good to leave a little mystery sometimes but eventually, it'll just get boring and the other party will distance themselves. Show that you are interested! It is perfectly okay.

Stay happy, the two of you enjoy yourselves and pay no attention to what anyone else has to say. The relationship only involves as many people as you allow.

15: To All of my Black Brothers and Sisters

Notice: I do not want any other race or ethnicity to feel discriminated against. That is not my intention. I have a duty to represent and give advice that I wish someone had given me as a young black woman. I am writing this book in a time where racism still exists and extreme colourism is at its peak and I can use the platform I have to address it. Everyone can, however, read it as it sends a message to every soul.

I am writing this chapter from experiences I have been through or realities around me. I cannot speak for any other race or ethnicity so not to misrepresent your reality. Feel free to read regardless because it may apply to you.

I know it can be hard to date when it has been said that black women (specifically darker skinned) are the least desirable. I disagree and many others do too. In fact, I don't actually know a man who wouldn't date a black woman. We have a lot to offer and anyone who says any different is a very confused individual. To let you beautiful, strong women know, we ARE desirable. There are men and women out there alike who love us despite our skin colour. In some cases, BECAUSE of our skin colour. Your skin colour, tone, and features, should never be insecurity of yours. Flaunt it! It is gorgeous and it makes you unique in your own right. You are beautiful, you are bold, you are powerful. Tell yourself this every day.

For all of my brown and dark-skinned women out there, love your melanin. Embrace everything you are. Let it pop. Wear whatever your heart desires! Bright colours and white look gorgeous on darker skin. Remember, the darker the berry, the sweeter the juice and it is no word of a lie. Black doesn't crack unless you do crack people!

Reminder: do not allow anyone to use you as a kind of fetish or something that they want to tick off from their twisted bucket list. We are worth more than that.

Some men and women absolutely love what we represent. They love our culture, our tendencies.

Do not allow for anyone to describe you as an 'angry black woman' or as aggressive because of your race. Any race can be angry. Any race can be aggressive. This is not a label that belongs to us, nor will it stick to who we are. There is absolutely nothing wrong with being opinionated. It is actually very beneficial to voice what your thoughts are and not allow just anyone to walk all over you. That is something that applies to absolutely every human being on the earth. You can pick the right moments to show submission. It can be as often or as little as you like. That decision is completely up to you and you should not be judged in a negative light for it.

If a man does not want you simply because you are black,

then guess what? It is his loss because we have a lot to give. Someone WILL appreciate that. Just be patient. Everyone has their individual preferences and do not be offended if you do not fall into that category. Some men or women prefer Caucasian women/men with blonde hair and blue eyes, some prefer brunettes. Some men or women prefer those who are biracial or Asian and guess what? There are more than enough men and women out there who prefer black women/men. As long as you are not being disrespected or insulted for who you are (things about yourself that cannot be changed) then there is absolutely nothing to worry about.

You yourself may have your own preferences and it is just the way life goes. I personally find it is beneficial for people to have an open mind and heart when it comes to dating but one cannot be forced into liking someone or something. Accept that fact and embrace those who embrace you.

There needs to be more of us, as black women and men **uplifting** each other. If we don't do it ourselves, then who will? If we as a collective are constantly bringing each other down then why is the next person going to respect us? No more spreading the hatred or the nasty comments. Remember where you come from. Your mother, sister, brother, aunties and uncles, grandparents and ancestors are black. Some of you will then have the temerity to negatively speak about a black woman because they're not as light as you'd like them to be? That is not right! It must stop. Nobody needs to change to be loved. As I keep repeating, there ARE men and women who will love a black woman and a black man unconditionally.

Pay no attention to those who use your race against you. You should pity them for their ignorance and their lack of integrity.

Everyone is entitled to have their preferences but never allow anybody to disrespect you. There is a line that should never be crossed and that is where I draw the line.

My boyfriend and I are of two different races. He is white and I am black but it has never mattered to him. He loves me for me and it truly is a beautiful feeling. If anything, the colour of my skin, the chocolate radiance, my sun-kissed glow, that all makes him crazy about me like I am about him. It goes deeper than just the colour of my skin. My culture, habits, traditions, and character all come into it in a positive way. He loves to learn more about me and I love to learn about him too. We both enrich one another's lives because of our differences. These qualities in us are what brought us together and what keeps us together. It is truly amazing to find someone who will embrace the person you are.

It is all about being open-minded. You may of course date outside of your race. Clearly, I am in support of that. However, **NEVER**, disrespect your black brother or sister because you are dating someone outside of your race.

If you are dating someone outside of your race, but have been raised in the same country, it may be easier for the two of you to get to know each other. You'll have a lot of cultural similarities. Use that to your advantage and make the most of it.

If you have not been raised in the same country/culture or you hold on to your culture/values that you grew up with a lot, then make sure you are with someone that is accepting, open-minded, interested in knowing more about you and even embracing it as their own too.

Never allow your race to be an obstacle to your relationship. The moment you feel ostracised then leave. Under no circumstances should you be subjected to any kind of hatred or poor choice of words from someone who doesn't appreciate you.

This chapter was to shed some light on what we as black men and women should be aware of. Nothing more, nothing less. We are all beautiful and we should love ourselves more than anyone can ever love us.

16: What it Takes to be a Successful Sugar Mum

Are you a sugar mummy looking for some good lovin'?

You're not sure if your sugar baby is with you for you or your money? Let me tell you this, though he/she may be with you for you, the benefits are also a part of it. It is part of being a sugar baby but just make sure that you are also being kept happy and you are not being taken for a fool.

Begin your sugar dating experience with a purpose. Do not charge in blindly. Make sure you roughly know what you are searching for in a partner and from the relationship because you could easily end up settling or falling for someone who is all wrong for you! Filter, filter, and filter the heck out of these searches when you are looking. Be choosy! It is your right! Just don't be unrealistically picky, that's when you'll find more issues.

Be confident! As a sugar mama you need to take charge and be assertive. You need to know what you are looking for in a woman or a man. There is no use of you being a sugar mama if you are going to allow someone to tell you how things are going to run (unless of course, that is your desire). It is up to you to take control and steer the relationship or arrangement your way. Go with the flow; move in the direction you want. Is it marriage? Is it a causal relationship? Is it just sex? Whatever it is, take your time to find it. Do not end up in any old lap. Make sure that the person you meet and are building something with is someone you can trust and be happy with, someone who is mature no matter how old they are. Just because they may be young enough to be your son does not mean that they will have a childish attitude. There are plenty of mature toy boys out there ladies! There are also plenty of mature and older men who would like to settle down again. Whatever you are looking for is out there.

Listen, some of you sugar mama's out there, you will be of a certain age, single with kids, maybe even married but not feeling like your husband is really fulfilling your needs so you are now looking elsewhere. Hey, I'm not here to judge. If this is the case, you may be feeling like a plain Jane. As if you just blend in with the wallpaper and only feel valued when something is asked of you. Well, let me tell you... YOU ARE ONE SEXY MAMA! Okay? Tell yourself every day in the mirror that you are one beautiful woman. Do not allow anyone to tell you otherwise. Just because you may be older does not mean you should let yourself go! Show you're sexy, be that woman, be the sexy, glamorous, rich, successful powerful woman that you are. Own your sh#t! You have absolutely nothing to lose and everything to gain!

To all you SMs' out there, life is too short. The last thing you should be doing is wasting your time. Do not play games or mess around with the man or woman you are dating. Ensure that dating him or her is something that you want otherwise you are wasting both of your time for no good reason. Do not waste or use the other person. They may not be as stable as you are and that is even more reason not to mess around with them emotionally or otherwise. Think carefully about what it is that you seek and would like to have in your life.

Now... the bitter truth is about to be told. Uh oh, right?

DO NOT BECOME EASILY LED OR USED.

Look... it is so easy to fall into the d#ck sand. I know, I know. I've fallen into my boyfriend's d#ck sand. However, when you barely know a person, it can become very dangerous.

A person can easily use and abuse you financially, physically and even emotionally can wear you down. You'll be broke and sad if you're not careful. Don't say I didn't warn you! I'm not saying this to put you off from ever taking care of the man that you are with, quite the contrary. Make sure you are handing over money, love, and sex to someone that has shown you their worth in your life. Not some gigolo or floozy. The man or woman you are with should show you he or she wants you in numerous ways. One of the more popular ways he/she can do that is intimately. A woman loves to feel desired so he/she should make you feel desired, cherished. Then you can spoil him or her however you want to! Do give him or her whatever you'd like. Just make sure you can tell the difference between someone who is genuine and a very good actor or actress.

What are you expecting from each other?

Make this clear when you are communicating. Would you like to be in financial control or should they participate?

Would you like to financially help them?

Are you going to be intimate?

Is there a possibility of commitment?

Is it an arrangement or relationship that suits you both?

Maybe they are even helping you with a particular struggle area in your life? For example, you need to go to the gym and you are now dating a personal trainer.

Are you adventurous? Are you kinky? Are they kinky? Are they open to trying out new things?

So many possible things to consider! It is all worth it once you find the right person.

A sugar mama will never follow the rules that were set out, rather she is a trailblazer who leaves her own path behind in order to chase the stars.

Sugar Mama Steps for Success

There's nothing wrong in admitting that you have no idea what you are doing. Do you have more questions than answers?

There. Doesn't that exposé make you feel much better?

Acknowledging that you are not sure what you are doing is the initial step towards a successful and fulfilling sugar mummy journey. Now I am going to help you take that next step to help you realise what you really want out of this experience.

Be impressive!

Take this very seriously! Don't be offensive and use proper grammar while speaking. Remember that if you are going to attract someone of worth, you have to be of high quality.

Always flesh out your profile.

If you do not say enough it will make you look suspicious. However, you need to leave some mystery as saying too much will be giving too much away.

Don't undermine the influence of words. Your profile tells a story. You want to tell a story and capture the attention of the right person. Your sugar mummy profile is **NOT** all about you. It's about capturing the mind of sugar babies you want.

Once you have got their attention, you will need to set up a date with your sugar baby. You need to focus on:

What are your goals?

What are you truly willing to invest in your sugar mummy

journey?

What are you going to do about it?

Try to avoid clichés.

Everyone around you thinks that they are the cleverest and most beautiful person on this planet. But what really is unique about you that makes you stand out?

Be modest, but try to find your niche.

You would probably know that all men are visual creatures so why no amuse them with a picture?

Car and bathroom shots aren't the best way to take pictures and I am guilty of this myself at times so please find someone who can take your full body shot which shows who you really are. Make sure your shots are recent and reflect who you really are.

I am aware of the fact that selfies are a trend but having different types of pictures in different locations, doing various activities will really capture part of your character.

Don't Forget How Fun and Hot You Are!

Being a sugar mama is an opportunity to be a different kind of 'you'. Before starting this journey, it's wise to get to know yourself. Well, this might sound a little vague, but it's actually quite simple. As a sugar mama, you are undoubtedly hot, fun and endlessly exciting. Always think about adding value to your life and to the lives of those around you – especially your sugar baby.

Communicate, Communicate, Communicate.

The whole reason why my relationship worked out was because we were honest and transparent with what we wanted from each other. Evaluate your needs and wants and put them on the table from the start. Your sugar baby will let you know what he/she wants from you and if you both agree, you'll get together.

Update your profile with what you want as it's the initial step in being direct. It is great to be straight about your demands but you also need to be accepting – Remember, it's all about getting mutual benefits.

Always be on the guard.

The real world is a scary place. So, when you are searching for a sugar baby, always keep in mind that there are bad apples among good ones. While using an online sugar dating website, remember to be careful and to verify all the potential babies.

Note: Check and double check that a potential sugar baby is telling the truth.

Trust your instincts.

Some nasty sugar babies can be extremely convincing. When you agree to meet him or her in private places, make sure that safety precautions have been taken and the necessary connections have been made.

We often see older females dating younger males nowadays in public. They will tell you upfront that they can give you good sex if you are interested but you must handsomely pay for their efforts and time. Most of them are even jobless and some of them don't even desire to be in a mutually beneficial relationship. They just want quick money with minimum efforts. **ENSURE THAT THEY MAKE AN EFFORT!** If they want to treat the arrangement like someone treats their job, make sure that they put the effort in to reap the rewards!

Demand Full Attention.

Remember that you are the one (most likely) with the busier schedule and job responsibilities. Your sugar baby should be bringing passion and a flexible schedule, which can easily work for you. I mean what is the point in keeping him or her around if he or she can't manage their time for you?

Sugar Alter: The Warning Signs.

If you are the one doing all the chasing.

If you are the one who is buying drinks and dinner ALL of the time – they should offer to at least pay out of courtesy a few times even if they know you will take care of the bill.

If you are the one using expensive gifts and money to induce a man/woman to spend time with you. By all means, treat your partner, spoil them even but **NEVER** buy their affection.

If you are the one trying to win the devotion of a sugar baby by paying for holidays and trips. Make sure your sugar baby is really into you before making such commitments. Do not book a holiday if they haven't invested themselves into the arrangement or the relationship.

<u>Remember</u>:

The way you are being in a relationship will determine the way the relationship is going to go. Don't assume you can change a month down the road, because you can't. Changing how you have been behaving/the agreement from the beginning will be the downfall of the relationship or arrangement. Unless of course you are upgrading something in the relationship.

Sugar babies feel happier and confident when they are in the company of their established sugar mummies. Besides offering financial stability, sugar mummies are kind, caring and they take good care of their sugar babies. They are provided with an extravagant lifestyle, frequent travel, good clothes and expensive gifts. Sugar Mummies are also sensational to be with (in and out of bed). They have experienced a lot in life, are ambitious and motivated, know what they really want and yet are still humble and aim to please.

It's no wonder that a **Sugar Mummy – Sugar Baby** relationship with younger males have been a hit. It sometimes develops into long-term relations and even perfect marriages.

Why do younger ladies look for sugar mamas?

Now have a look at why younger ladies are look for sugar mamas.

'**Comfort**' again is the key reason. Women-to-Women, Lady-to-Lady – there is so much that a sugar mummy and her female sugar baby have in common.

Needs wants, lifestyle and interests tend to be the same. And of the same gender; they can clearly understand each other. A **Sugar Mama – Sugar Baby** pair makes for a great companionship, sexual intimacy, and romance.

Some character traits of sugar mamas

-       Strong
-       Independent woman
-       The female force which keeps going with determination
-       Takes accountability for her comfort
-       Laughs at herself when needed
-       Loves herself and plays to win

17: LGBTQ Community

I couldn't write a book about dating without addressing the LGBTQ community directly! I won't dive into a long paragraph because I'm a heterosexual female and I can't speak on the struggles you may face daily but still, I'd like to give some words of encouragement.

So here it goes...

For some of you, more than others in this community, you may find it more challenging to openly date or find someone who is accepting of who you are.

Well, it shouldn't be that way. Everyone should have an opportunity to date who they want and be accepted no matter what! I haven't got much to say because there shouldn't be anything said in the first place! You are no alien and should be treated like any heterosexual person.

Embrace who you are, love who you are no matter how the next person may make you feel. You have no reason to be ashamed of who you are because some people don't view life the way you do.

Date who you want to, it is easy to also date on sugar dating websites. Quite a few of them give you open options when signing up so it'll be easier for you to find those you are attracted to and those who are also attracted to you!

I hope that you give sugar dating a try because more and more individuals are becoming open and honest about who they are meaning more people for you to date!

Hopefully, I can shed some light about being a sugar baby in the LGBTQ world and how to approach this.

There is a common misconception among being bisexual. People say that the minds are 50% liking men and 50% liking women. Well, that might be true for some of you but the way I see it is that sexuality is a scale which varies. Somebody could need women more than men and feel reverse of that the next day or even years far along. There is nothing wrong about this because that is what a person's mind or heart desires. Our society is now grown to accept that same sex relations are just as human as the opposite.

Remember that you are not defined by your sexuality.

Whether you are confident in who you like, it is your time to begin dating.

If you have made up your mind to dip into the sugar bowl, it's vital to know that what you are up against. Let's begin with gay sugar baby tips:

Gay Sugar Baby Tips.

If you have decided to begin the journey to become a gay sugar baby, there is surely a likelihood of attaining a nice income and an extravagant lifestyle, but it can take a fair bit of effort.

- **Understand what you want:** It's important to figure out what it is you want exactly. Are you expecting a regular income or travel and adventure? Or you could be looking for someone to guide you and help you succeed in your chosen career. Whatever it is, it's important to be REALLY clear about what you want.
- **Set the terms:** After finding a good match, clarify your hopes with your sugar daddy as soon as possible. Keep in mind that it would be wise to wait until after your first meeting. You are exchanging the boyfriend experience here, you don't want to come across as a gold digger.
- **Be a good listener:** It is important to make eye contact, don't interrupt or jump to conclusions. Let him know that you are hearing what he has to say.
- **Offer to pay – Both of You:** Both of you belong to the same sex, and until you have agreed on the term for who pays for what, you both should offer to pay.
- **Communicate:** Now that you have found your gem amongst the pebbles, you definitely don't want to lose him. Drop them texts asking if there's something they need from you. Don't Lie.
- **Mentor him:** Guide him and lead him down a trail he has shown interest in for his career. Even if you are eager to provide for your Gay Sugar Baby for all of their life, this might not be what they want.

Tips on How to Find a Gay Sugar Baby

- Do a little bit of research.

- Set the rules.

- Play by the rules you have set.

- Have fun.

Here I will need to split up the sexes:

Women: Resist the urge to merge. Don't U-HAUL for at least a year. It's a recipe for disaster.

Men: Label it. Call it what it is. If you desire an open relation, clearly express it to your partners; likewise; if you desire a monogamous relationship then express. In case you are somewhat in the middle – clarify that too.

For a perfect moment, you need to give it a try! You will get to know when the moment is right.

Anyone who has given a chance to a mature man can tell you exactly how much these sophisticated gents have to offer – they are established, ambitious and have the balance you need in your life. If you are a young guy searching for a sugar daddy, then there are so many dating websites out there where you can meet these well-established gay sugar daddies who appreciate the spontaneity of young men and prefer their company. If you feel you are of the type and yearn for a successful sugar daddy to compliment you in life, then register yourself on the dating site and make a compelling profile that will help you find a potential sugar daddy to breathe some fire into your love life!

How to become a successful Bisexual or Lesbian Sugar Baby

Usually, when we think about sugar dating, we think about an old rich man providing for a hot and sexy young woman. But that doesn't mean that lesbians are left out of the equation. Surely, there is a romantic and sexual dimension to sugar mama dating. I am listing some steps to help you figure out whether sugar dating is an option for you – irrespective of your sexual orientation.

Ever been with a man before?

Not everyone is 100% gay or straight. If men don't repulse you physically and you really want to be a sugar baby, then by all means, GO FOR IT. Find a sugar daddy who appeals to you and who you genuinely like and attracted to.

Be straight about who you are.

It isn't right to hide who you are. It will just make things worse and hard for you if you don't disclose it in the first place. If you stay open from the start, you stand a chance of finding an open-minded sugar daddy or mummy who will be more turned on by you. **Take full benefit of the fact that you are different.**

You can still have a girlfriend.

Being a sugar baby doesn't mean that you can't date or have a girlfriend. Chances are that you won't have to hide this fact from your sugar daddy or mummy either. If you are upfront then you can have the best of both worlds. Many sugar daddies and mummies out there like to have a third person involved in the mix.

You can leave anytime.

You aren't bound into a lifelong commitment. You can pull the cord anytime and get out if you decide that sugar dating isn't for you. Give it a shot, and choose wisely. Give it your best but if things don't work out, you don't need to feel bad. **Cut your losses and move on.**

You might find a sugar mama.

Yes, they are out there. Often, you need to hunt for those ladies. You will definitely find them if you look for them. Sugar mummies are rich ladies who want to spoil some hot young girls for fun. If you are sexy and determined enough, you too can find your very own. **Or maybe they will find you.**

Listen, Listen, Listen.

On your first date, when you are getting to know each other, listen closely. Women have a lot to say, use a lot of words and get into the details – it's all important to most women. Let her do most of the talking. You will learn tons about her that you need to know.

As I have mentioned before, that not everyone feels comfortable being upfront in their profile. You may not essentially wish to keep this a secret, but might prefer to disclose it in a private conversation. It takes a lot of courage for LGBT people to be open and honest – **So be respectful if they choose to confide in you.**

You shouldn't feel bad for wanting to pursue a relationship. Just be sure to express your true feelings.

It's easy to rush into dating, into sex, and into commitment. But it never helps anyone when it comes to LBGT dating. Take your time to get to know someone. Being thoughtful means that you have spent time looking back on your life and figured what could work and what couldn't in your relationship.

Now get yourself ready for dating.

Well, if you are going do it online, then use **GREAT** pictures of yourself. It means a really good shot with a **SMILE** on your face really visible. Get online and search dating websites, things will definitely pop up.

Often in case of Transgenders, some people fail to understand them at first but they are just like anyone else and shouldn't be treated otherwise.

<u>Always do what works for you</u>

The decision is always yours whether or not to disclose your identity. But think about the positive things which can happen only when you are upfront with who you are. Also, if you are to date someone, it is a must to disclose your sexuality to them should they not know. They have a right to know so they can make their decision accordingly. Mention it to yourself, make yourself safer and more comfortable. It is your unique point and something special which helps you stand out of the crowd. **Value it and find a sugar daddy or mummy who values it too.**

18: ENJOY! Have Fun!

There's not much else to say apart from enjoy and cherish every moment you spend with your other half. There is a whole world out there to explore! Free your mind, body, soul and spirit. Do whatever you each decide in a judgement free zone!

There is no shame in having fun with someone older/younger, different, wiser, successful. It is part of how we develop further and enable growth. Go on that trip, create new memories together and start new adventures.

Pay no mind to those who have anything negative to say because no amount of negativity should impact your life. Especially if the negativity comes from someone who benefits you in no way or plays no significant role in your life.

The world is your oyster. Life is what you make it. Living la Vida loca. All of these sayings could be what your life represents. No need to be stressed or take life too seriously. Live in the fast lane! Have your fun. I really can't stress that enough. Life is too short to be stressing over the small stuff. Having someone around can really help to take any worries away and just make you feel safe, secure, like it is just the two of you. Spending time with your partner can make it feel like nobody else exists and you just feel happy. Nothing else matters.

Change your routine, upgrade your life and network. Even if it doesn't work out as a relationship, dating can be fun. You can even make great friends along the way. It is a good way to socialise and branch out. One date could change your life for the better.

19: The Website - RichMeetBeautiful®

This chapter may be one that you have all been waiting for, the website.

RichMeetBeautiful® is an online sugar dating network for both men and women over the age of 18 that seek a mutually beneficial relationship.

I found my amazing man on RichMeetBeautiful®. Now, I am not saying that this website will work for everyone because no website does but it did for me and so, I have got to recommend it to anyone who is trying to find their 'one'.

This website has members from all over the world! You can communicate with the SD/SM for free if they are to approach you first so ladies (and men), get those hot pictures up!

The website encourages anyone who joins to find exactly what they're looking for. The aim is to fulfil each other's wants and needs and that is exactly what this website and those who have joined can and will offer. Listen, you only live once so don't think too hard about this one!

You can gain so much more in life by just meeting the right person. You can shape your future, set your lifetime goals, you'll be able to just be open and honest with one another and feel comfortable with that. This is a zone where everyone can just speak their minds (respectfully of course). The two (or more) of you can set your own conditions, make your own rules or have absolutely no rules! It can be whatever you'd like it to be and that is the beauty of it.

You will experience so much joy, have many adventures and be filled with passion! A healthy and balanced relationship is exactly what RichMeetBeautiful® can offer to anyone who joins. There is someone out there for everyone and all you have got to do is open that door.

The Last Chapter: Safety Tips

I know, I know. The end already? I'm afraid so folks.

I have given all the broad advice that I can give without knowing specific individual situations but do not worry, you won't be left high and dry. There are other ways to get more specific advice from me! Just reach out to me and I will be happy to help.

I couldn't write this book without giving any safety tips and warnings. The most important thing to remember when dating, especially online dating is to stay safe.

Staying safe should be on your mind at ALL times and can vary from when you begin to talk to someone, when you meet them, when you are intimate to even travelling together for the first time.

There are a few things to remember;

<u>Early stages of getting to know each other/planning to meet:</u>

-   Ask questions. There is nothing wrong with being nosey when getting to know someone. As long as it is nothing too personal, you have the green light when it comes to asking questions.
-   Exchange pictures. Even when there are pictures on a

profile, it is important to exchange a few more in different settings. It helps to get to establish what kind of a person they are.

- Speak on the phone. Phone calls or video calls are crucial. You should never meet anyone without doing one of the two or both. It helps to put a voice to the face and is a great way of establishing some trust.
- Do not send money (unless it is part of the 'deal'). It just isn't safe especially when there are scammers online.
- Planning to meet. Set a specific time and destination so there are no grey areas.
- Decide whether or not you are being picked up/picking up/meeting at a certain place. Be careful about giving your full address. Maybe give a nearby road and walk over to the pickup point.
- Be yourself. You have no reason to put up a front. It'll show very soon.

Meeting the person;

- Meet in a public place. It's crucial that the two of you feel safe when meeting. Should anything go wrong, you can easily escape and have the public around you. Go for a hot drink or to a bar. Try to avoid a hotel on the first date.
- Aim for good timing. A nice lunch is good for getting to know each other. I'd say dinner and drinks is more for when the two of you feel comfortable with each other as it is more of a relaxed setting.

- Come up with different date ideas. The old-fashioned ideas are okay but testing the waters doing different activities can never do any harm. Go to the zoo, an aquarium, do a hobby that you both enjoy together and bond.
- Ask personal questions. At this stage, you have established that you like each other enough to meet in person. So, ask away! Set the mood, then ease in with the questions.
- Take extra money for an emergency (in case anything goes wrong) and keep your phone charged!
- Keep the same energy you had when you first began to talk. Do not become a bore.
- Men, do not be a pervert. Do not come across as sleazy and desperate. Do not lead with sex. Even if your arrangement is about sex.
- Women, do not lead with money talks, do not go on and on all night about what you expect from him or what your ex did.
- Establish what the two of you expect from each other. Discuss it in less than five minutes and move on from it, then go from there. It'll either be something you're okay with or something you're not okay with.
- Do not talk about ex's or present partners unless it comes up. It is just about the two of you.

Intimacy:

- Condoms. Use them. Pregnancy and STDs/STIs are

real and can be very inconvenient not to mention a health hazard. If the two of you decide not to use them, make sure you are in the all clear health wise, are monogamous and that the woman is using some sort of contraception unless of course, you are trying for a baby.

- Mark your boundaries. Talk about what you are okay and not okay doing or being done to you.
- Do not become intimate without establishing trust.
- Hygiene. This goes without saying but you'd be surprised so make sure all genitals are well taken care of and the body is smelling fresh.

Travelling:

- Have a copy of all of your holiday details. You'll need to let someone know some of the details (flight, hotel).
- Double check that everything is in order. Travelling with no organisation or certainty is not recommended.
- Know who you are travelling with. Don't know their surname? Don't go.
- Have some money reserved in case of an emergency and you need to catch a flight back home.
- Have an itinerary when going on holiday so the days are not wasted away.
- Pack smart. Do not overload your suitcase with unnecessary items. Pack as light as you can because you may even go shopping at some point.
- Do not leave your luggage in the hands of anyone but your own. Building that trust between you before that

can happen is important.
- Keep the atmosphere between the two of you good.
Having bad vibes when you're away can be toxic and
awkward.

Long story short, vet the person you will be spending your
time with, do not be naïve when it comes to dating. Keep
your eyes open and stay vigilant! Do not place everyone in
the same pot. Not everyone out there is a disappointment.
Enjoy yourself, have some carefree fun and feel guiltfree.

Overall, I am hoping that you have picked up a thing or two
and will take it on board and put it to action. Feel free to
send me a message if you have a question! Avoid asking
questions that have been answered in the book because
I'll send you right back to it! I will be answering any
specific questions you may have that the book has not
directly addressed or any nerve calming you may require. I
am at your service.

Now go and LIVE LIFE IN THE FAST LANE!

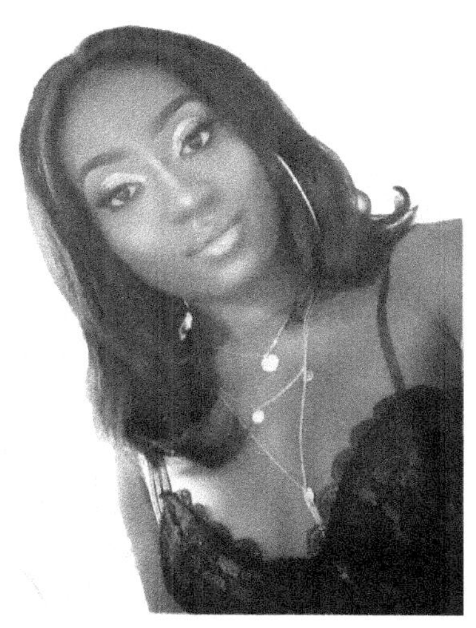

Stephany Alleyroux

www.ingramcontent.com/pod-product-compliance
Lightning Source LLC
Chambersburg PA
CBHW050007070726
47592CB00018B/1077